Clinical
Atlas of
Peripheral
Retinal Disorders

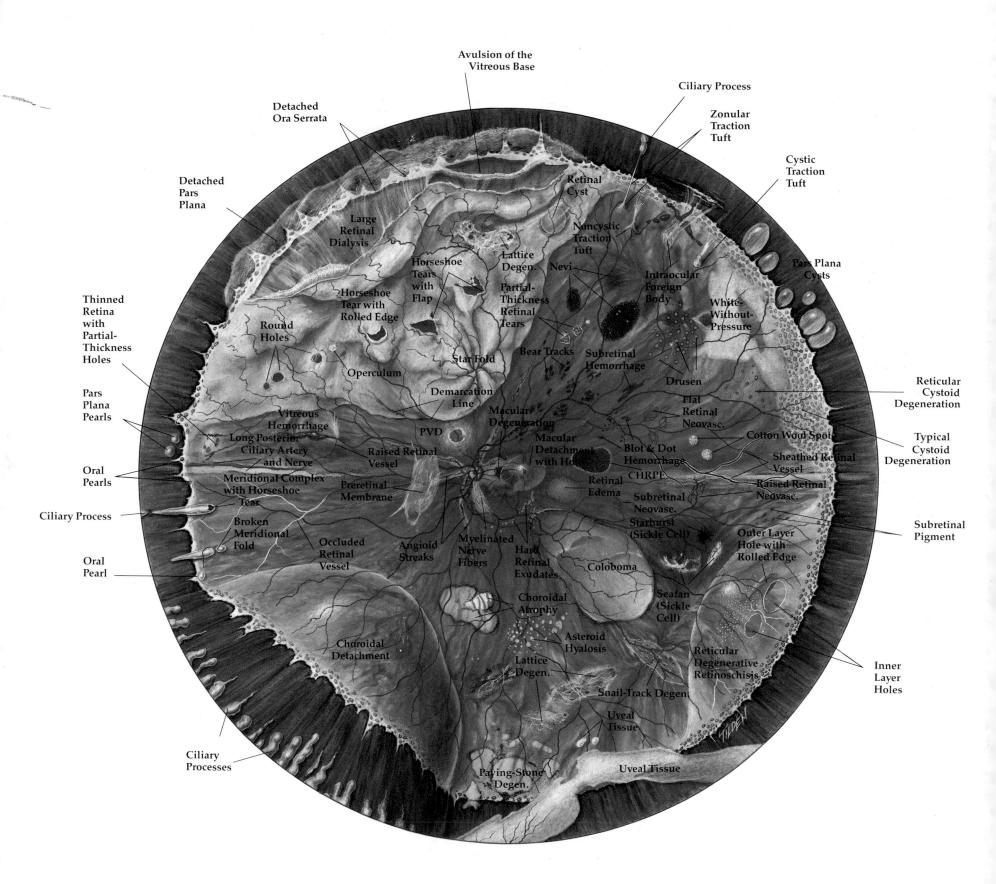

Composite Fundus Pathology

Clinical
Atlas of
Peripheral
Retinal Disorders

Keith M. Zinn

Clinical Professor
Department of Ophthalmology
Mount Sinai School of Medicine
New York, NY 10029

Attending Ophthalmic Surgeon
Manhattan Eye, Ear, and Throat Hospital
New York, NY 10021

Illustrated by

David A. Tilden

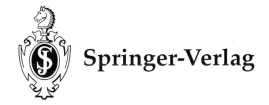

Springer-Verlag

Keith M. Zinn, M. D.
Clinical Professor
Department of Ophthalmology
Mount Sinai School of Medicine
New York, NY 10029, USA

Attending Ophthalmic Surgeon
Manhattan Eye, Ear, and Throat Hospital
New York, NY 10021, USA

Illustrator
David Anders Tilden
Active Member: Association of Medical Illustrators
Active Member: Guild of Natural Science Illustrators
44 Wirt Way
Duxbury, MA 02332, USA

Cover Illustration
Congenital Hereditary Retinoschisis
(Juvenile Retinoschisis [Fundus]) (Plate 28)

Library of Congress Cataloging-in-Publication Data
Zinn, Keith M., 1940–
    Clinical atlas of peripheral retinal disorders.
    Bibliography: p.
    Includes index.
    1. Retina-Diseases-Atlases. I. Title.
[DNLM: 1. Retinal Diseases-atlases. WW 17 Z78c]
RE551.Z56   1988   617.7′3   88-6536
ISBN 0-387-96459-2

Typeset, printed, and bound by H. Stürtz AG, Würzburg, Federal Republic of Germany.
Printed in the Federal Republic of Germany.

9 8 7 6 5 4 3 2 1

ISBN 0-387-96459-2 Springer-Verlag New York Berlin Heidelberg
ISBN 3-540-96459-2 Springer-Verlag Berlin Heidelberg New York

To the memory of my father Victor Zinn. His love of life and knowledge was an inspiration for all those who were fortunate to know him.

Leon Hess, a wonderful friend, for his many years of brotherly advice and encouragement.

Robert Heidell, Esquire, for his wise counsel.

Irving H. Leopold, M. D.: a great clinician, teacher, and chief.

Charles L. Schepens, M. D.: a superb ophthalmic surgeon and innovator, without whom this book would not have been possible.

Contents

Chapter 7
Degenerative Conditions of the Vitreous Body   73

Chapter 8
Proliferative Retinopathies   79

Chapter 9
Inflammatory Disorders   89

List of Plates

Preface

A comprehensive understanding of diseases of the peripheral retina is essential to the general ophthalmologist as well as to the vitreoretinal surgeon. Expertise in indirect ophthalmoscopy, scleral depression, and contact lens biomicroscopy serves as a basis for observing the peripheral retina. These observations are then recorded on fundus drawing paper and the Tolentino vitreo-retinal chart. This orderly sequence of skills allows the ophthalmic surgeon to objectively diagnose and evaluate specific peripheral retinal disorders and plan for their therapeutic management.

The *Clinical Atlas of Peripheral Retinal Disorders* is a compilation of fundus paintings by David A. Tilden based on our observations of a large number of patients over the past 15 years. The atlas is organized along functional and anatomical lines. After a brief introduction to the clinical anatomy of the peripheral retina, the appearance of the fundus as a function of skin color and aging is presented. Many of the diseases of the peripheral retina can be divided into trophic (nutritional), tractional, and a combination of trophic plus tractional etiologies. This classification system, although somewhat simplistic, appears adequate for our present level of understanding of the pathogenetic mechanisms of these disorders. Undoubtedly, once the molecular biology of these conditions is elucidated through future research, the classification will be revised. In addition, there are other conditions that affect the peripheral retina that do not fit the proposed classification system and are covered under separate headings, i.e., congenital defects, neoplasms, metabolic disorders, etc.

The *Clinical Atlas of Peripheral Retinal Disorders* is not meant to be an encyclopedic treatise on the subject, but rather a compendium of the more significant peripheral retinal diseases that befall the human condition. The Bibliography is more of a suggested reading list for those interested in gaining more detailed knowledge of specific retinal disorders.

The fundus color code appears in Chapter 14. Alongside each code item is the way it would be drawn by the ophthalmologist and the way it would appear in the actual fundus painting.

The *Clinical Atlas of Peripheral Retinal Disorders* is meant for residents, fellows, and ophthalmologists in general practice as well as for vitreoretinal surgeons. The goal of this atlas is to impart an understanding of disease patterns affecting the peripheral retina which will aid in arriving at the correct diagnosis and successful management of these disorders.

I am indebted to my teacher, Dr. Charles L. Schepens of the Harvard Medical School and The Retina Foundation in Boston, for his tireless efforts to instill in me the skills of indirect ophthalmoscopy with accurate observation of ocular pathology which is the basis for this Atlas. Many of the observations in this book are a direct result of Dr. Schepen's brilliant work as a surgeon and innovator over the past four decades. I am also indebted to the following superb individuals who were my teachers at The Retina Service of the Massachusetts Eye and Ear Infirmary and The Retina Foundation: Drs. R.J. Brochurst, H. McKenzie Freeman, T. Hirose, W. McMeel, I. Okamura, R. Pruett, and C. Regan.

I would like to thank David A. Tilden, medical illustrator extraordinaire, for his tireless efforts in portraying the fundus paintings which are at the heart of this

Atlas. Mr. Tilden has pioneered many illustration techniques in the area of fundus paintings over the past 20 to 25 years that are reflected in the artwork in the book.

Grateful acknowledgement goes to Barbara Goldman, Editor at Springer-Verlag, for her organizational spirit and drive which was essential in publishing this Atlas. In addition, I'd like to thank the publishers, Springer-Verlag, for their kind help and advice in publishing the Atlas.

Keith M. Zinn, M.D., F.A.C.S.

Anatomic Considerations   1

The Vitreous

The vitreous is a unique tissue in that it is transparent, allowing for the transmission of light entering the eye and eventually reaching the neurosensory retina. The vitreous has other unique properties in that it is avascular at birth and has viscoelastic properties that allow it to act as a shock absorber, dampening mechanical vibrations that might affect the retina. Yet the vitreous is 99% water and the remaining 1% is made up of special collagen fibers and hyaluronic acid molecules. The normal vitreous has certain immunologic properties as well as the ability to inhibit neovascularization. In short, the physical and chemical properties of the vitreous are most unique and unlike that of any other collection of extracellular material in the body.

In the adult, the volume of the vitreous ranges between 3.5 and 3.9 ml and comprises 66 to 75% of the total volume of the globe. The vitreous body has a spherical shape posteriorly with a saucer-shaped indentation anteriorly where it is in contact with the posterior surface of the lens. The outermost layer of the vitreous is termed the cortex and is divided into an anterior cortex region and a posterior cortex region by the vitreous base. The vitreous base is a zone of cortical adhesion varying between 2 and 3 mm in width, straddling the ora serrata region of the peripheral retina and running for 360°.

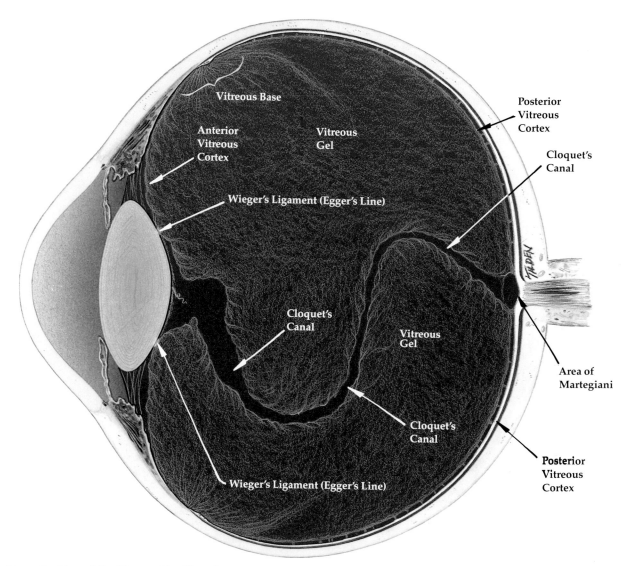

**Cross Section of the Human Eye Showing
Cortical Zones and Vitreous Base**

Vitreous Attachments to Intraocular Structures

Anterior Vitreous Cortex

The anterior vitreous cortex is in intimate contact with the ciliary body and the posterior surface of the lens. The circular line of adhesion of the anterior vitreous cortex to the posterior surface of the lens is termed *Wieger's ligament* and has a diameter of about 8 mm. Although the term Wieger's ligament is widely used for this adhesion, it is not a true ligament.

In young individuals, under the age of 40 years, Wieger's ligament has a fairly strong connection to the posterior lens capsule, but as an individual approaches 40 years, this ligamentous adhesion dissipates and is almost inconsequential. Because of the strong Wieger's ligament attachment forces in young people, intracapsular cataract surgery is usually not possible without loss of vitreous and therefore extracapsular cataract surgery is carried out. In older patients, intracapsular cataract surgery can be carried out with relative ease once Wieger's ligamentous attachments to the posterior lens capsule have become minimal. Alpha-chymotrypsin has no dissolving effect on Wieger's ligament.

Modern cataract surgery with posterior chamber intraocular lens implants is almost always performed using the extracapsular extraction technique. This provides an intact posterior lens capsule which serves as a physical barrier preventing the anterior vitreous from prolapsing into the anterior chamber. This has resulted in a dramatic reduction in the incidence of retinal detachments postoperatively.

Vitreous Base

The region with the strongest attachment of the vitreous to the inner wall of the globe is the vitreous base, which is a zone of attachment that is 2 to 3 mm wide and straddles the ora serrata region, running parallel to the equator for 360°. The vitreous base extends 1.0 to 1.5 mm anterior to as well as posterior to the ora serrata (see Plate 8, p. 14). When vitreoretinal tractional forces are created in the vitreous base region, these forces can often lead to retinal tears, retinal dialyses, and even disinsertion of the vitreous base. The anterior and posterior borders of the vitreous base can be seen in most patients using peripheral indirect ophthalmoscopy with scleral depression.

Posterior Vitreous Cortex

In general, the posterior cortex of the vitreous normally is adherent to the inner surface of the retina. The posterior vitreous cortex has several important connections to the inner surface of the retina in the peripapillary and macular regions. The posterior vitreous cortex is not attached to the surface of the optic nerve head, but only at its edges, and these attachments are termed the peripapillary connections. In addition, there are attachments along major retinal vessels called paravascular connections. There is a mild but variable adhesion of the posterior vitreous cortex to the macula with stronger attachments to the inner surface of the retina in the equatorial region. When there is a complete posterior cortical vitreous detachment, the peripapillary vitreous attachments also detach. Since they are usually translucent, they cast a shadow when there is light falling on the retina and are perceived by the individual as "floaters." Occasionally, a small peripapillary hemorrhage or a vitreous hemorrhage may take place as a result of a posterior cortical vitreous detachment. In certain cases, where an abnormal vitreoretinal adhesion exists, a posterior cortical vitreous detachment can lead to a retinal tear and possibly to a rhegmatogenous retinal detachment.

Vitreous Attachments to Intraocular Structures Plate 2

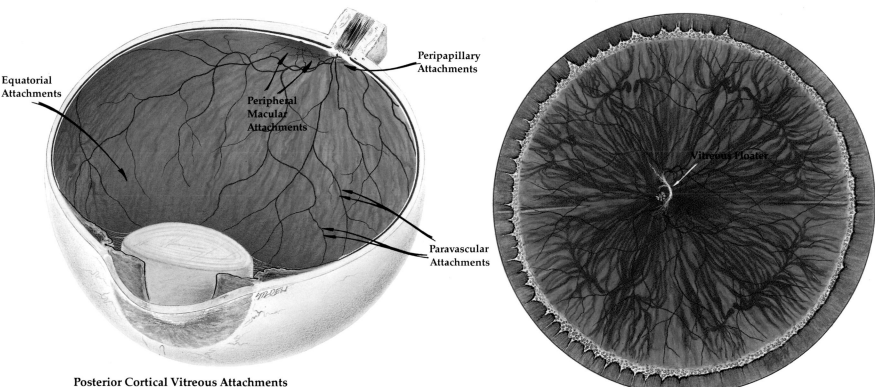

Equatorial Attachments

Peripheral Macular Attachments

Peripapillary Attachments

Paravascular Attachments

Posterior Cortical Vitreous Attachments to the Optic Nerve Head and Retinal Tissues

Vitreous Floater

Simple Posterior Cortical Vitreous Detachment – Full Fundus

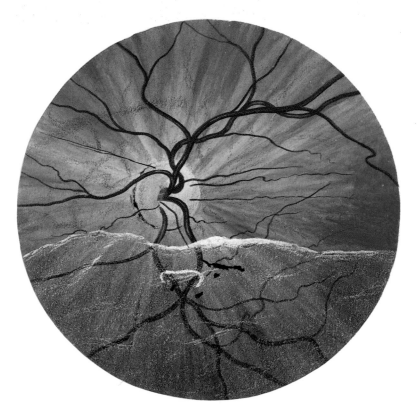

Simple Posterior Cortical Vitreous Detachment – Posterior Pole

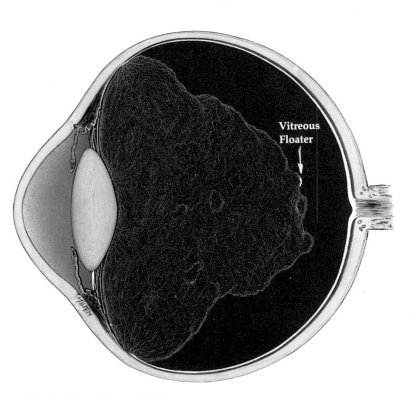

Vitreous Floater

Simple Posterior Cortical Vitreous Detachment – Cross Section

Plate 3   **Anterior Cortical Vitreous Canals and Spaces**

Vitreous Canals and Spaces

Petit's canal is a potential space in the retrolenticular region peripheral to Wieger's ligament and is actually an interface between the anterior vitreous cortex and the inner surface of the zonules and posterior lens capsule. *Berger's space* is a retrolenticular space within the *circular line of Egger* and is bounded anteriorly by the anterior vitreous cortex and posteriorly by plicated vitreous membranes in the anterior expansion of *Cloquet's canal*. *The space of Erggelet* is a retrolenticular space that is part of the anterior expansion of Cloquet's canal and found just below the visual axis. Berger's space is only one portion of the much longer space of Erggelet. Patients with uveitis, vitreous hemorrhage, and retinal detachment may have cells in Berger's space that can be detected with slit-lamp biomicroscopy.

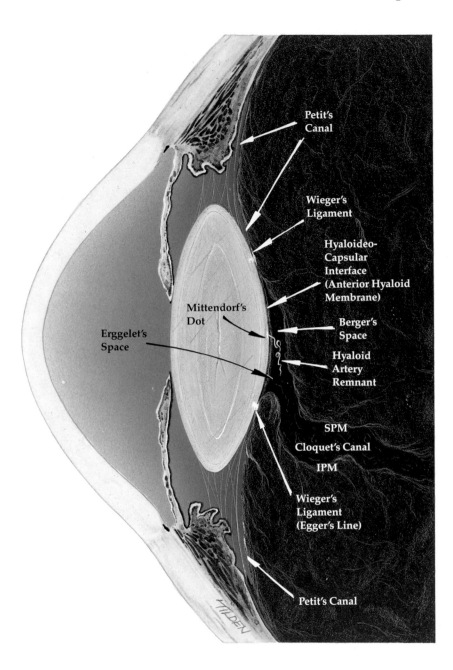

IPM = Inferior Plicated Membrane
SPM = Superior Plicated Membrane

In phakic patients, without a history of ocular inflammation or surgery, one may see pigment cells or "tobacco dust" in the anterior vitreous cortex region, which is termed *Shafer's sign*. The pigment granules in this case may represent dislodged retinal pigment epithelium that entered the vitreous cavity through a retinal tear site. Therefore, Shafer's sign, when noted on biomicroscopy, should alert the examiner to the possibility of a retinal tear or a possible retinal detachment in the eye.

The *central hyaloideocapsular space* is a potential space that is actually an interface between the anterior vitreous cortex and posterior lens capsule. This interface opens when the anterior hyaloid and the posterior lens capsule are separated mechanically. It has been noted to be open in eyes with an anterior vitreous detachment associated with Marfan's syndrome and in cases of ocular trauma.

Cloquet's canal is an undulating tubular structure that courses through the vitreous body from the optic disc to the patellar fossa. The anterior and posterior ends of Cloquet's canal are expanded to form the space of Erggelet and the *area of Martegiani*, respectively. The lumen of Cloquet's canal is quite variable, but is narrowest in the midvitreous. During embryologic development, Cloquet's canal contains the hyaloid vascular system.

Shafer's Sign   **Plate 4**

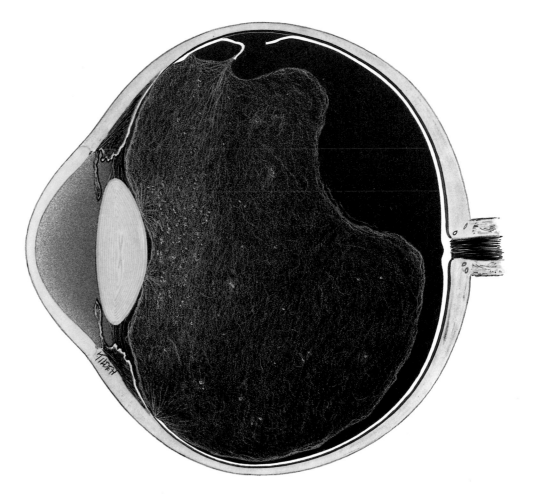

Anatomic Nomenclature of the Fundus

When clinicians view the fundus with various instruments, the peripheral fundus is divided into hemispheres and further subdivided into quadrants, as depicted in Plate 5. In addition, a clock with its hour markings is superimposed upon the fundus of each eye and is used as a frame of reference for specific lesion sites. For example, a retinal tear is located at the 2:30 o'clock meridian near the equator, or a retinal detachment involves the inferonasal quadrant.

Localization of lesions is thus recorded using this coordinate system of clock hours, and frontal plane landmarks such as the equator, vortex vein ampullae, and the ora serrata region.

Anatomic Nomenclature of the Fundus   **Plate 5**

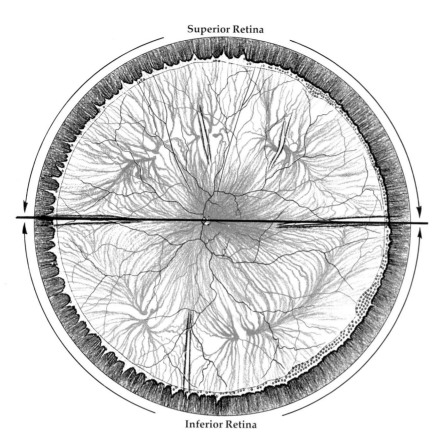

Superior Retina

Inferior Retina

Superior Half and Inferior Half of the Retina (Fundus)

Superonasal

Superotemporal

Inferonasal

Inferotemporal

Temporal and Nasal Quadrants of the Retina of the Left Eye (Fundus)

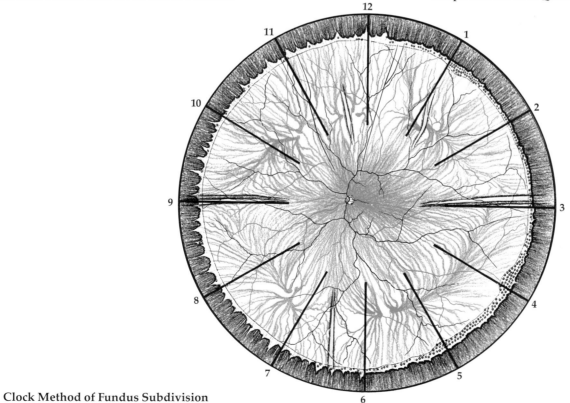

Clock Method of Fundus Subdivision

The Neurosensory Retina

The neurosensory retina extends from the edges of the optic nervehead to the ora serrata, after which there is a single layer of nonpigmented epithelium covering the pars plana. The neurosensory retina is strongly anchored at the edges of the optic nervehead and at the ora serrata region. This retinal attachment is strongest temporally where the pigment band at the ora serrata is widest (1.5 to 2.0 mm). Nasally, the pigment band is narrowest and is therefore weakest. The nasal ora serrata tends to be scalloped with fine toothlike projections of retina onto the pars plana termed *dentate processes*. Regions between neighboring dentate processes are called *ora bays*. In addition, there is a weaker adhesion of the neurosensory retina to the subjacent retinal pigment epithelium. When a retinal detachment occurs, the neurosensory retina detaches from the retinal pigment epithelium and loses some of its normal transparency.

The retinal vessels are located in the innermost surface of the retina (closest to the vitreous) and diminish in their cross-sectional diameter as they branch out from the optic disc toward the retinal periphery. Normally, the last 1 to 2 mm of peripheral retina at the ora serrata region tends to be avascular. The retinal arterioles are brighter red and of smaller caliber compared to retinal veins at a given distance from the optic nervehead.

The macular region, 0.22 mm thick, is the thickest portion of the neurosensory retina, except for the foveal pit, which is about 0.10 mm thick. The peripheral retina is about 0.12 mm thick. The macula is darker in color than the surrounding retina because of the carotenoid pigment xanthophyll glycol located in the outer plexiform layer of Henle and because of the increased number of pigment granules in the taller retinal pigment epithelium cells within the macular region. In contrast, the extramacular regions do not have any appreciable carotenoid pigment and have flatter retinal pigment epithelium containing less pigment (melanin) granules.

The Choroid

The retinal pigment epithelium and the choroid provide nutrition to the outer one third of the neurosensory retina and also provide a pump that is responsible for the basic adhesive force of the neurosensory retina to the retinal pigment epithelium. The choroid extends from the optic nerve head peripherally to the ora serrata region and is strongly anchored to the optic nerve head and to the scleral tissue at vortex vein exit sites. Anteriorly, the choroid is continuous with the pars plana of the ciliary body. Elsewhere, the choroid is clearly adherent to the sclera by means of a loose matrix of suprachoroidal tissue.

Ophthalmoscopically, there are three basic morphologic patterns of the choroid that should be appreciated: (1) the choroidal pigment pattern, (2) vortex vein systems, and (3) choroidal landmarks.

Choroidal Pigmentary Pattern

The pigmentary color pattern one sees in a patient will depend upon a variety of factors, such as the amount of pigment in the retinal pigment epithelium cells and in the branched melanocytes within the choroidal stroma as well as the density and thickness of the choroidal stroma and vascular system. The choroidal pigment is densest in the suprachoroidal space and poorest where large choroidal vessels are present, especially in the vertical meridians.

As a rule, the choroid is thickest in the posterior polar region where the choroidal pigmentary pattern is less distinct. The choroidal pigment does not always correlate with the pigment of the hair, skin, and irides. However, an albinotic fundus would be lighter than a fundus in a blond person, which in turn would be expected to be lighter than in a brunette or a Negro. One could arrange ocular fundi in an order from light to dark color as follows: albinotic, blond, brunette, Asian, Mediterranean, and Negro. It is important to note that there are variations of fundus color among each of the different races. The fundus color will also vary with the age of the individual.

Choroidal sclerosis of the blood vessels makes the vessels stand out, but aging changes in the retinal pigment epithelium, for example, in senile macular degeneration, may obscure the underlying choroidal pattern.

Vortex Venous System

The choroidal veins drain the choroidal tissue as well as the anterior segment and form whirl-shaped tributaries that ultimately flow into a larger vein known as the *vortex vein*, which exits from the eye through a scleral canal. Approximately 50% of the vortex veins in normal eyes have an aneurysmal dilation termed the *ampulla*, into which the tributary veins empty, and then the blood leaves the eye via the vortex vein. Most vortex veins are near the equator. There is usually one vortex vein per quadrant, which tends to be located at or near the 2, 4, 8, and 10 o'clock meridians. The vortex veins in the superior quadrants drain into the cavernous sinus, whereas the vortex veins in the inferior quadrants drain into the cavernous sinus or enter the external jugular vein via the pterygoid plexus that passes through the inferior orbital fissure.

Vortex vein ampullae have a wide variety of anatomic configurations and on occasion can be seen to pulsate spontaneously, or when pressure is applied to the globe, or when the eye is rotated in such a position that the superior oblique muscle can open the intrascleral canals. This allows rapid emptying of blood from the ampulla into the vortex vein and out of the orbit.

The Fundus   **Plate 6**

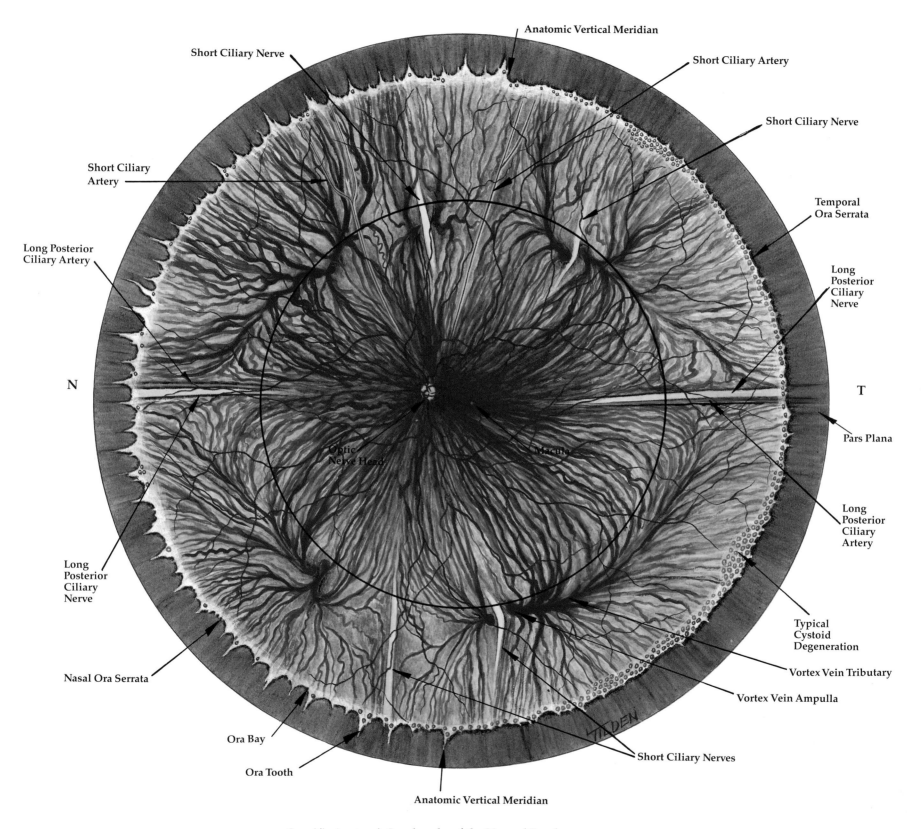

Specific Anatomic Landmarks of the Normal Fundus

Obstruction of a vortex vein leads to a choroidal hemorrhage. If several vortex veins are obstructed simultaneously, a variety of sequelae may take place as follows: choroidal hemorrhage, subretinal, retinal, and vitreous hemorrhage, glaucoma, anterior segment ischemia (corneal edema, corneal vascularization, corneal ulcers, anterior uveitis, peripheral anterior and posterior iris synechiae, iris atrophy, iris neovascularization, neovascular glaucoma, ocular hypotony, cataract, and phthisis bulbi). Therefore damage to vortex veins is to be avoided whenever possible in retinal detachment and orbital surgery.

Choroidal Landmarks

The fundus can be divided into quadrants, using choroidal landmarks. The long posterior ciliary arteries and nerves found at the 3 and 9 o'clock meridians serve as the horizontal meridional landmarks. The short ciliary nerves and arteries located near the 6 and 12 o'clock meridians serve more or less as the vertical meridional boundaries.

The *long posterior ciliary artery* is a bright, thin, red line in the horizontal meridian with some pigment in its adventitial wall that is seen ophthalmoscopically beginning in the posterior segment, extending peripherally to the ora serrata and pars plana region. The long posterior ciliary artery usually runs a straight course in the fundus and rarely branches. The long posterior ciliary artery will anastomose with the short ciliary arteries to form the *vasculosis iridis major* located in the ciliary body. The long posterior ciliary arteries and the short ciliary arteries form the blood supply to the anterior segment of the globe.

The *long posterior ciliary nerve* usually runs with the long posterior ciliary artery in the fundus at the horizontal meridian; it has a flat appearance, rather like a linguine noodle. The nerve has a pigmented epineurium, which helps to define its edges and make it more easily visible on ophthalmoscopy. The long posterior ciliary nerve is first seen in the horizontal meridians near the posterior segment, then extends peripherally to the ora serrata and pars plana regions and does not usually branch along this route. The long posterior ciliary nerve conducts pain and temperature information from the anterior segment back to the gasserian (trigeminal) ganglion of the Vth cranial nerve.

The long posterior ciliary artery and nerve run side by side in the fundus at the choroidal level. Nasally, the long posterior ciliary artery is superior to the long ciliary nerve, and temporally the long ciliary nerve is superior to the long posterior ciliary artery.

Damage to the long posterior ciliary artery and nerve, for example, as in scleral buckling surgery, may lead to anterior segment ischemia and obviously is to be avoided. Transillumination of the globe during retinal detachment surgery leads to easy identification of the long posterior ciliary artery and nerve so they can be avoided when diathermizing a scleral bed.

In many fundi, the long posterior ciliary artery and nerve are easily noted on ophthalmoscopy, but in a number of fundi one or more of the structures cannot be seen because of pigmentary choroidal patterns. However, it has been estimated that, in 95% of fundi, one or more long posterior ciliary arteries or nerves will be visible in the fundus periphery near the horizontal meridians.

The *short ciliary arteries* tend to be located near the vertical meridians and are twice as numerous near the 6 o'clock meridian than near the 12 o'clock meridian. Also, the choroid is poorly vascularized near the vertical as well as the horizontal meridians.

The anterior short ciliary arteries are derived from the vessels on the rectus muscles, which pierce the globe at the insertion points of the rectus muscles. The anterior short ciliary arteries join the long posterior ciliary arteries in the ciliary body to form the *vasculosis iridis major* (circulus arteriosus major).

The *short ciliary nerves* are smaller than, but similar in appearance to, the long posterior ciliary nerves. The short ciliary nerves are more often visible inferiorly at or near the 6 o'clock meridian. They enter the globe posteriorly after leaving the ciliary ganglion. They run anteriorly with the ciliary arteries, innervate the ciliary body, iris, and cornea, and send pain and temperature information from the anterior segment back to the central nervous system. The short ciliary nerves also carry efferent sympathetic fibers to the iris dilator muscles and efferent inhibitory sympathetic fibers to the iris sphincter and ciliary body musculature.

Equator

The *equator* of the globe has been defined as that region of the eye where a frontal plane intersecting the globe gives the greatest cross-sectional diameter. The equator of the globe has no specific landmarks and is variable, depending upon the size and shape of the eye. The equator is usually located 2 disc diameters anterior to the circle intersecting the scleral entrances of the vortex veins' ampullae. The vortex veins are located in the equatorial region. The scleral exit sites of the vortex veins are located more posterior to the limbus in the superior quadrants (20–21 mm), as compared to the inferior quadrants (17–18 mm).

The peripheral retina is further divided up equally between the equator and the ora serrata into an anterior zone (anterior half) and a posterior zone (posterior half) by an imaginary line that is parallel to the plane of the equator. This imaginary line is equidistant between the ora serrata and the equator.

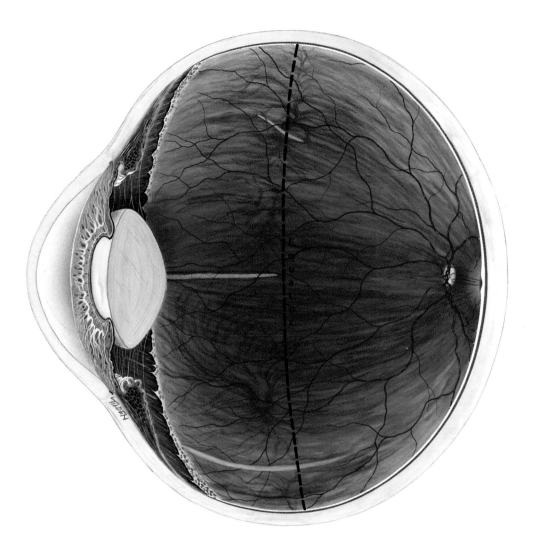

Plate 8   **Three-Dimensional Cutaway View of the Ciliary Body and Ora Serrata Region**

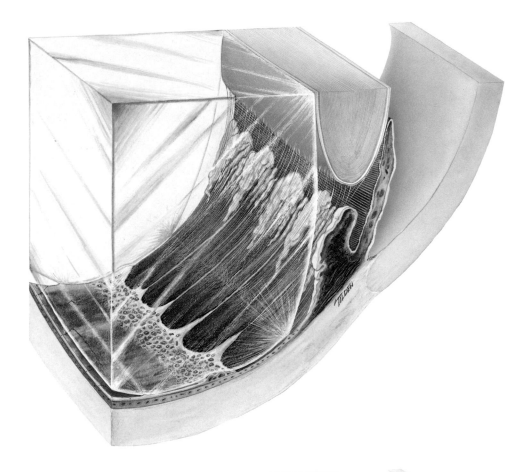

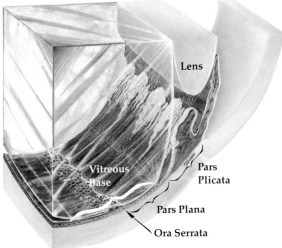

Pars Plana

The ciliary body is divided into an anterior portion termed the *pars plicata* and a posterior portion termed the *pars plana*. The pars plana is 4 mm in its radial length, extending from the ora serrata anteriorly to the posterior edge of the pars plicata. The pars plana is relatively avascular and therefore is the preferred site for pars plana vitrectomy incisions and for intraocular injections; it is also the choice site for removal of small intravitreal foreign bodies. The majority of lens zonules insert in the valleys between pars plicata processes, but on occasion the lens zonules can anchor in the pars plana region and can even connect with the fibers of the vitreous base. Occasionally, tears in the nonpigmented epithelium of the pars plana may lead to retinal detachments. Cysts of the pars plana usually involve the nonpigmented epithelial layer and are benign. In multiple myeloma, the cysts contain myeloma protein.

Pars Plicata

The pars plicata is the anterior portion of the ciliary body and there is an average of 70 pars plicata processes per eye. Each process is approximately 2 mm in length and is the source of aqueous humor. The zonular fibers of the lens are inserted in the equatorial region of the lens capsule and are anchored in the valleys between pars plicata processes. In some eyes, the zonules continue posteriorly and insert into the anterior portion of the vitreous base meshwork. Because of this relationship, it is possible during cataract surgery to generate retinal breaks at the posterior border of the vitreous base. Excessive tractional forces on the lens capsule during surgery appears to be the responsible mechanism.

Ora Serrata

The anterior or peripheral edge of the neurosensory retina is termed the *ora serrata*. Typically, the temporal portion of the ora serrata tends to be smooth. In the nasal half of the ora serrata there are frequent projections of neurosensory retina onto the pars plana. These retinal projections have been likened to teeth, hence the term *dentate processes*. Areas between adjacent dentate processes are known as *ora bays*. On occasion, one can find smooth regions of the ora serrata nasally and the dentate processes temporally. In some eyes, adjacent dentate processes meet and are fused, forming an *enclosed ora bay*, which can be mistaken for a peripheral retinal hole. Also, there is more pigment along the ora serrata nasally than temporally, with greater adhesion of the nasal retina to the underlying choroid.

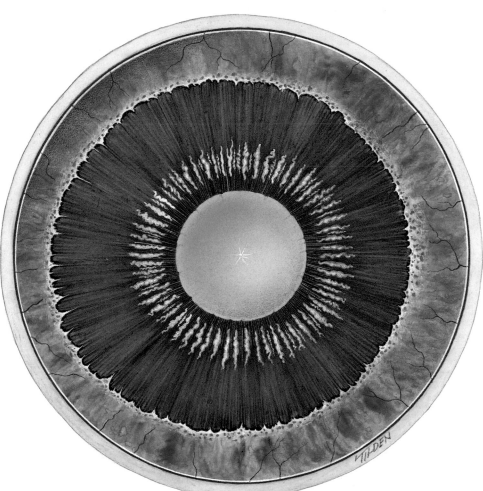

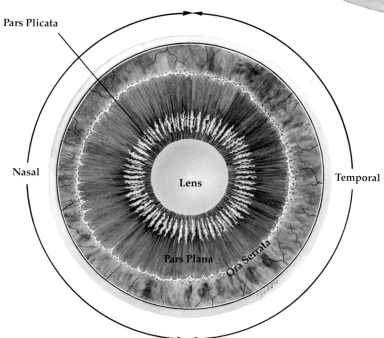

Variations of Fundus Appearance

Fundus Appearance as a Function of Aging
In the infant fundus, there is a wet silk appearance to the inner surface of the retina. The retinal periphery is almost devoid of dentate processes, in contrast to the adult. Therefore, ora bays are not seen, except in some cases where there are bifid dentate processes. Also, there is no cystoid degeneration, and the pars plana is almost nonexistent. More specifically, the ora serrata almost abuts the posterior aspect of the pars plicata processes.

As the individual ages and the eye grows in size, dentate processes, ora bays, and a distinct pars plana are established. After the age of 20 years, typical peripheral cystoid degeneration is almost a universal finding. With aging, there are cystic changes in the retinal periphery, as well as chorioretinal degeneration and atrophy, as outlined in Table 1.1. Many of these changes reflect alterations in the retinal and choroidal circulations and the mechanical wear and tear caused by motion of the vitreous base in response to eye movements and body movements.

Each of these aging features is discussed in detail in separate sections of the atlas, classified along specific anatomic lines.

Table 1.1.

Aging Changes in the Peripheral Fundus

Cystoid changes
　　Typical cystoid degeneration
　　Typical degenerative retinoschisis (acquired)
　　Pars plana cysts

Chorioretinal degeneration
　　Honeycomb degeneration
　　Equatorial drusen
　　White-without-pressure

Chorioretinal atrophy
　　Paving-stone degeneration

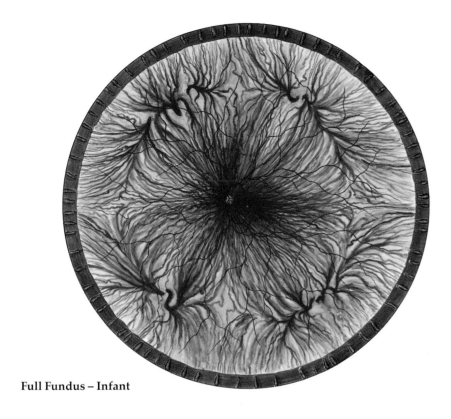

Full Fundus – Infant

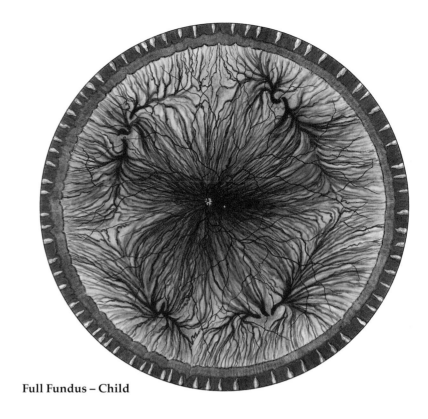

Full Fundus – Child

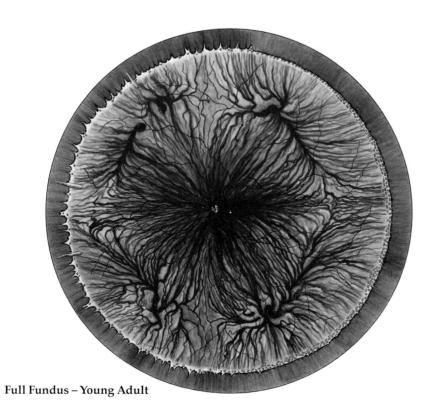

Full Fundus – Young Adult

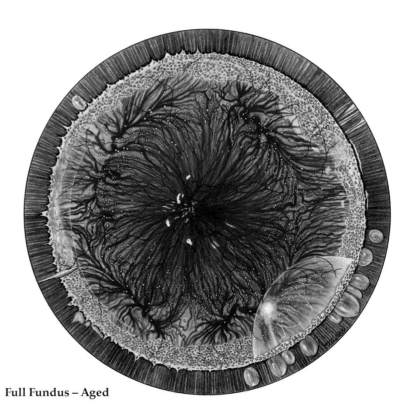

Full Fundus – Aged

Plate 11   **Pars Plana Cysts**

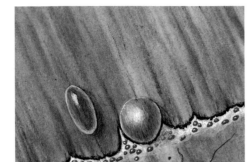

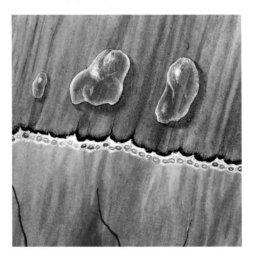

Pars Plana Cysts
Another cystic aging change occurs in the pars plana and is known as the pars plana cyst. Pars plana cysts are round or oval transparent elevations of the nonpigmented epithelium of the pars plana and contain hyaluronic acid. They represent cystoid spaces between the nonpigmented and pigmented epithelium of the pars plana. In some patients with macroglobulinemias and dysproteinemia, for example, multiple myeloma, the cysts have a slightly turbid appearance because they contain abnormal proteins. Although there does not appear to be a specific relationship of pars plana cysts with other ocular pathology, they are believed to be more frequent in patients with retinal detachments.

In general, pars plana cysts range in size from 0.25 to 2.5 disc diameters and have the appearance of a translucent grape. They are often found in the temporal quadrants of adult eyes. Pars plana cysts are more readily apparent on indirect ophthalmoscopy and scleral depression and appear to be located in the posterior half of the pars plana. There is no particular sexual predilection. In persons over 40 years old, 24% have at least one pars plana cyst, and in 33% of these cases the cysts are bilateral.

Fundus Appearance as a Function of Body Pigmentation
There is a wide variation found in the pigmentation patterns of the normal fundus, which appears to be correlated, in most cases, with the skin pigmentation of the individual. It is also important to recognize that within a given skin pigmentation category, there will be a wide spectrum of fundus color.

Albino
There is little pigment within the choroidal melanocytes, which is responsible for the light-colored appearance of the fundus and for the prominence of the choroidal vascular pattern.

Blond
The blond fundus has more pigment in the choroidal tissues than an albinotic fundus, but less than that of a brunette.

Brunette
Moderate amounts of pigment in the choroid give the brunette fundus an appearance that is darker than that of the blond fundus. The greater concentration of choroidal pigment tends to obscure some of the choroidal vascular pattern.

Asian
A heavy concentration of pigment in the choroidal tissues of Asians often masks the choroidal vessels, hindering visualization on ophthalmoscopy. Geographic white-without-pressure may be seen in the retinal periphery and also posterior to the equator.

Negro
In the Negro there is perhaps the greatest concentration of pigment in the choroid among all skin colors, which also makes visualization of the choroidal vessels somewhat difficult. There are often areas of geographic white-without-pressure anterior to, as well as posterior to, the equator.

Variations of Fundus Appearance as   **Plate 12**
Function of Body Pigmentation

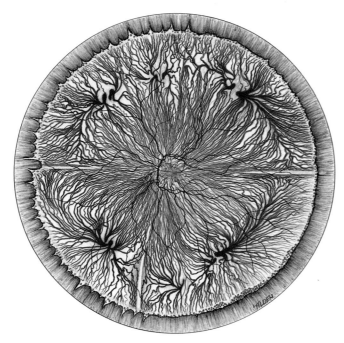

Albino

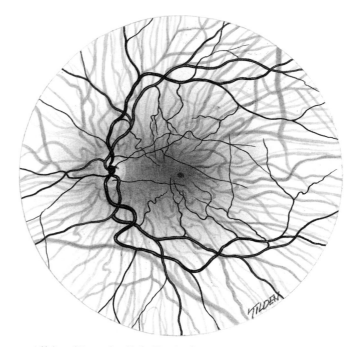

Albino (Posterior Pole Region)

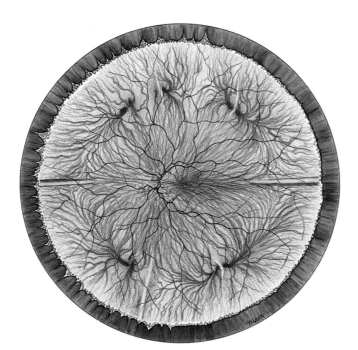

Blond

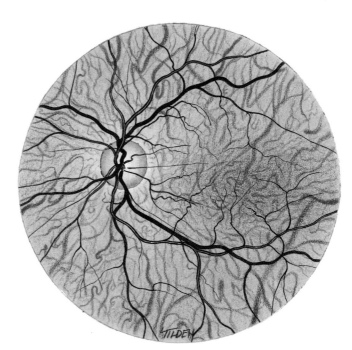

Blond (Posterior Pole Region)

Plate 12   **Variations of Fundus Appearance as
                        Function of Body Pigmentation**

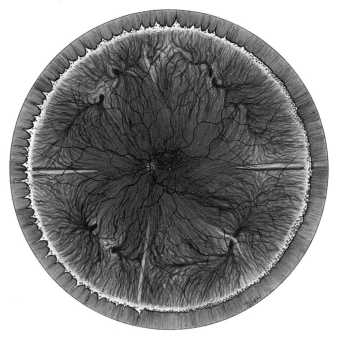

Brunette

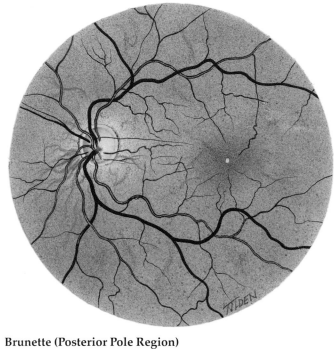

Brunette (Posterior Pole Region)

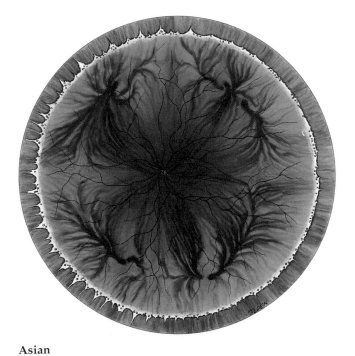

Asian

Asian (Posterior Pole Region)

Variations of Fundus Appearance as   **Plate 12**
Function of Body Pigmentation

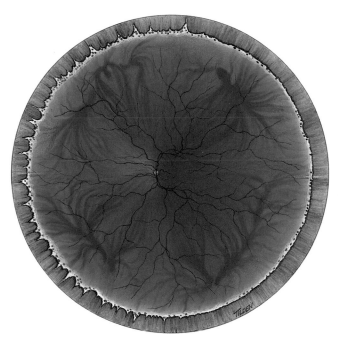

Negro

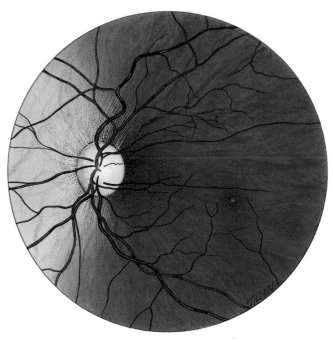

Negro (Posterior Pole Region)

Fundus Appearance as a Function of Refractive Error

Hyperopic and emmetropic fundi do not have specific peripheral retinal changes as related to the refractive error of the eye. However, the myopic eye tends to have a number of fundus changes, depending upon a number of factors including the magnitude of the myopia. These myopic fundus changes are summarized in Table 1.2.

Table 1.2.
Myopia Fundus Characteristics
Temporal tilting of optic nerve head
Peripapillary choroidal atrophy
Myopic macular degeneration   Fuchs' spot
Posterior staphyloma
White-without-pressure
White-with-pressure
Lighter choroidal pigmentation

Larger eyes
  ↑ Anteroposterior diameter
  ↑ Cross-sectional diameter

Wider pars plana

Variations of Fundus Appearance as   **Plate 13**
Function of Refractive Error

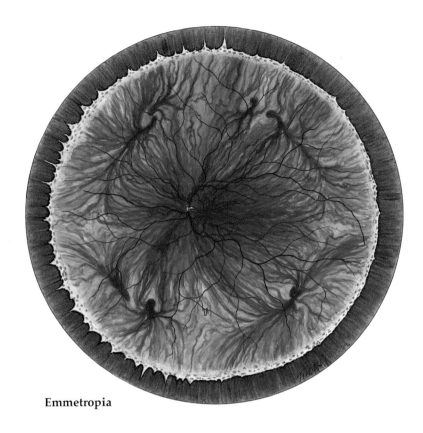

Emmetropia

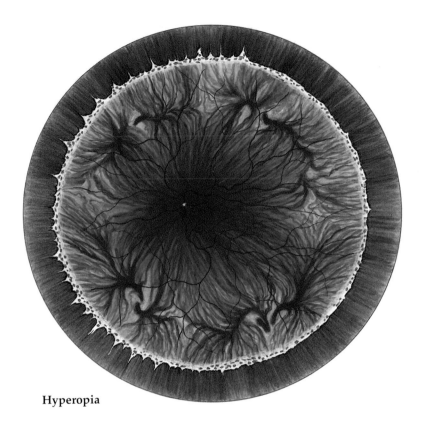

Hyperopia

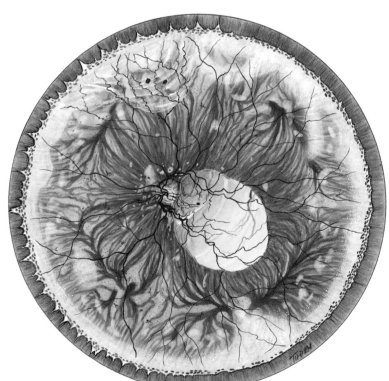

Myopia (Full Fundus View)

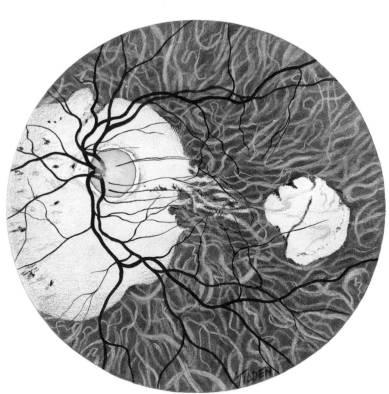

Myopia (Posterior Pole View)

Classification System of Peripheral Retinal Degenerations 2

Developmental variations refer to anatomic variances in the peripheral retina that are most likely embryologic in origin. *Peripheral retinal degenerations* represent alterations in previously normal retinal structures as a result of either a *trophic* (nutritional and/or vascular) or a *tractional* disturbance. In some degenerations, there are trophic as well as tractional factors responsible for the pathogenesis of the lesion, for example, lattice retinal degeneration.

It is interesting to note that retinal breaks can have a trophic and/or a tractional origin. When a retinal break is due to tractional forces then it is termed a *retinal tear*. Otherwise the term *retinal hole* is used to describe a break of trophic (nontractional) origin. In some cases, trophic and tractional elements combine to produce a retinal break. Because of the presence of tractional forces, it is termed retinal tear.

Since the pathogenesis of most of the peripheral retinal disorders is not known, a relatively simple classification has been devised by a number of authorities based on presumed etiologic factors and is outlined in Table 2.1. As our knowledge of these diseases improves, undoubtedly this classification system will be replaced.

Table 2.1.

Classification of Peripheral Retinal Developmental Variations and Degenerations

Developmental variations

Peripheral retinal degenerations
  Trophic
  Tractional
  Trophic ⊕ tractional

Developmental Variations of the Peripheral Fundus   3

Generally, at least one developmental variation of the peripheral retina is present in 20 to 47% of all eyes. Developmental variations have the following features: they are present at birth, persist throughout life, have mirror symmetry between the two eyes, and often have an associated dentate-ciliary process alignment abnormality in the same quadrant as the developmental variation. The developmental variations are listed in Table 3.1.

Variations of Ora Serrata Bays and Teeth

Over 30% of normal eyes will show at least one of the following developmental variations: giant ora bays, giant dentate processes, bridging teeth, bifid teeth, or ring teeth. These variations tend to be located in the horizontal meridians over or near the long posterior ciliary artery and nerve.

Ora Bays
Deep ora bays are at least sixfold more common than any other ora serrata developmental variation and tend to be bilateral. A deep bay is from two to four times wider and deeper than neighboring ora bays. As a rule, the dentate processes bordering a deep ora bay are longer than nearby tooth processes.

Giant Teeth
Giant ora teeth are wider and longer than the average dentate process and extend into the anterior portion of the pars plana, and in some cases are contiguous with the posterior aspect of a pars plicata process. Giant teeth are found in association with deep ora bays and are the most frequent developmental variation of teeth found, yet they are not as common as deep ora bays.

Bridging Teeth
A bridging oral tooth is a cordlike extension of peripheral retina that arches over the ora serrata and pars plana and inserts in the anterior portion of the pars plana and is not associated with the lens zonules as is a zonular traction tuft.

Ring Teeth
Two adjacent dentate processes can fuse anteriorly in the pars plana creating an *enclosed ora bay*, which may be mistaken for a retinal break. There are different stages of ring teeth, for example, open, partially closed, and completely closed.

Bifid Teeth
Bifid teeth have a fork-shaped appearance and are slightly larger than the usual dentate process and are common in infant eyes.

Table 3.1.

Developmental Variations of the Peripheral Fundus

Variations of ora bays
  Deep or giant bays
  Partially enclosed bays
  Enclosed bays

Variations of ora teeth
  Giant teeth
  Bridging teeth
  Ring teeth
  Bifurcated teeth (bifid)

Meridional folds
  Bay folds
  Tooth folds
  Complexes

Granular tissue
  Noncystic tuft
  Cystic tuft (granular globule)
  Zonular traction tuft

Ora serrata pearls

Meridional Folds

Meridional folds are radial pleats of peripheral neurosensory retina underlying the vitreous base, measuring 0.5 to 1.5 disc diameters in length and 0.3 disc diameters in elevation. The meridional folds tend to be translucent and often show cystoid degeneration. The overlying vitreous and subjacent retinal pigment epithelium appear to be grossly normal, yet, on histologic examination, loss of outer and inner segments of photoreceptor cells is evident.

Meridional folds are associated with dentate processes 70% of the time and are termed *tooth folds* or *dentate folds*. The remaining 30% of meridional folds are associated with ora bays and are termed *bay folds*. A meridional fold aligned with a dentate fold, contiguous with an enlarged ciliary process, is termed a *meridional complex*. About 61% of all dentate folds are part of a meridional complex, and 27% of these have an associated thinning of the retina at the posterior border of the meridional fold. In some cases, this progresses to a retinal tear or hole, which may eventually form a retinal detachment.

The incidence of meridional folds is 26% of all eyes after the age of one year and is bilateral in 48% of cases. Single meridional folds in an eye occur 68% of the time, whereas 32% of cases have from two to six meridional folds per eye. There is a predilection (86%) of meridional folds for the horizontal meridians, especially on the nasal side.

Variations of Ora Serrata Bays, Teeth, and Meridional Folds   **Plate 14**

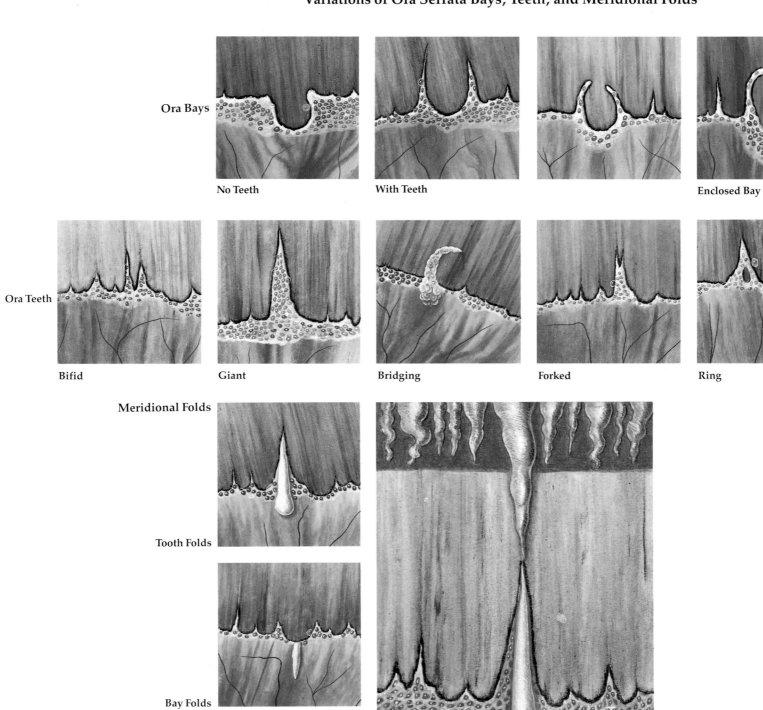

Ora Bays

No Teeth

With Teeth

Enclosed Bay

Ora Teeth

Bifid

Giant

Bridging

Forked

Ring

Meridional Folds

Tooth Folds

Bay Folds

Broken Tooth Fold

Meridional Complex

Granular Tissue (Tufts)

Granular tissue consists of fine elevations, tufts, or projections of neurosensory retina arising from its inner (vitreal) surface. Granular tissue is usually found in the retinal periphery, mostly on the nasal side. Histologically, it contains elements of proliferated and degenerated neurosensory retina along with normal retinal tissue. Granular tissue (noncystic, cystic, zonular) comes in a variety of shapes and configurations, which will be discussed below. In general, granular tissue does not change in size, number, or distribution within an eye during the life of the individual and is not usually associated with retinal tears or detachments.

Noncystic Retinal Tuft (Granular Tag)

A noncystic retinal tuft or granular tag is a thin, short, internal projection of retinal tissue, usually located within the posterior portion of the vitreous base with a vitreous attachment at its apex. The tuft is composed of altered retinal cells and proliferated glial tissue. The base of the tuft is usually less than 0.1 mm in diameter, and the underlying retinal pigment epithelium is normal. The incidence of noncystic retinal tufts is 72%, and is bilateral in 50% of cases. One tuft occurs in 36% of eyes, and 64% of the remaining eyes have from two to six tufts per eye. Noncystic retinal tufts tend to be found in the inferonasal quadrant and are not, as a rule, associated with retinal breaks.

Cystic Retinal Tuft (Granular Globule, Patch)

A cystic retinal tuft consists of a plaque, globule, or nodule of peripheral retinal tissue that projects into the vitreous body. It is composed of degenerated cystic retinal tissue and proliferated glial elements. Its shape is variable, but it does have a base that is greater than 0.1 mm in diameter and is larger than a noncystic retinal tuft. Cystic retinal tufts are usually located within the vitreous base region and posterior to a meridional fold.

Cystoid degeneration is found in this type of cystic retinal tuft, and condensed vitreous bands are often visible at the apex of the tuft. Occasionally, dispersed pigment granules are present in the underlying retinal pigment epithelium.

Cystic retinal tufts are found in 59% of eyes, and of those cases 39% are bilateral. In the affected eyes, 35% have one cystic retinal tuft, and in the remaining 65%, 2 to 7 tufts per eye can be found. There is a predilection for the superonasal quadrants, and 96% of cystic retinal tufts are located underneath the vitreous base. Cystic retinal tufts are rarely associated with retinal breaks.

Zonular Traction Tufts

Zonular traction tufts are peripheral retinal projections extending anteriorly over the pars plana, whose apex is attached to one or more thickened zonular fibers. The tufts originate immediately posterior to the ora serrata and contain variable amounts of cystic degeneration, pigmentation, retinal thinning, and gliosis. Zonular traction tufts are larger and longer than the cystic and noncystic retinal tufts, and, in contrast to these other tufts, retinal breaks may occur at the base of the tuft.

The incidence of zonular traction tufts is 16%, and is bilateral in 11% of cases. About 66% of affected eyes have one zonular traction tuft per eye, and the remaining 34% of cases have multiple tufts per eye. Zonular traction tufts have a predilection for the inferonasal quadrant.

Ora Serrata Pearls

Ora serrata pearls are pinpoint-sized, round, glistening, yellow-white, sometimes calcified structures located on dentate processes, the pars plana, or on peripheral retina near the ora serrata region. Most ora pearls are located on a dentate process and a few are located on an ora bay. Ora pearls have a predilection for the superotemporal quadrant and the horizontal meridians. Histologically, the pearls are similar in appearance to *drusen* and have acid carbohydrate staining properties. The pathologic significance, if any, of ora serrata pearls is not known. They are believed to be of developmental origin and are found in 20% of adult eyes.

Granular Tissue (Tufts) and Ora Serrata Pearls

Plate 15

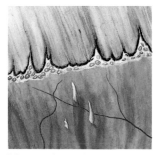

Noncystic Retinal Tuft (Tag)

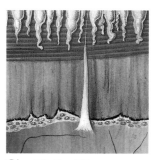

Giant Retinal Tag

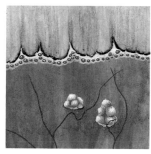

Cystic Retinal Tuft

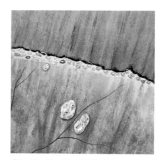

Cystic Retinal Tuft (Granular Tissue)

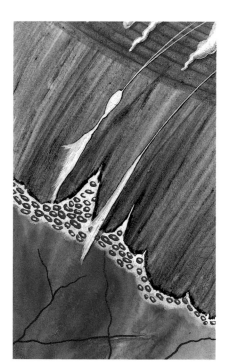

Zonular Traction Tufts

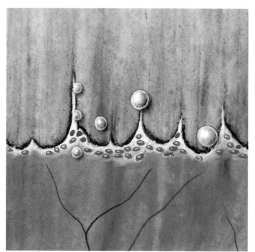

Ora Serrata Pearls

Trophic Retinal Degenerations 4

Inner Neurosensory Layer
   Vitreous Base Excavations
   Retinal Holes

Middle Neurosensory Layer
   Typical Cystoid Degeneration
   Reticular Cystoid Degeneration
   Acquired Typical Degenerative Retinoschisis
   Reticular Degenerative Retinoschisis

Outer Neurosensory Layer – Retinal Pigment Epithelium
   Paving-Stone (Cobblestone) Degeneration
   Peripheral Tapetochoroidal (Honeycomb) Degeneration
   Equatorial Drusen

Trophic retinal degenerations are characterized by some vascular, metabolic, or nutritional disturbance as the main pathogenic mechanism.

It is useful to divide the peripheral neurosensory retina (nonpigmented) into three separate layers, each about one-third of the thickness of the retina. Thus, there would be an inner (nearest to the vitreous), a middle, and an outer (nearest to the retinal pigment epithelium) neurosensory layer. This artificial separation of the neurosensory retina into layers is a helpful device in classifying and understanding trophic and tractional retinal degenerations. The trophic disturbances are classified along regional anatomic lines in Table 4.1.

Table 4.1.
Trophic Retinal Degenerations

Inner neurosensory layer
    Vitreous base excavations
    Retinal holes (partial, complete)

Middle neurosensory layer
    Typical cystoid degeneration
    Reticular cystoid degeneration
    Acquired typical degenerative retinoschisis
    Reticular degenerative retinoschisis

Outer neurosensory layer – retinal pigment epithelium
    Paving-stone (cobblestone) degeneration
    Peripheral tapetochoroidal
        (honeycomb) degeneration
    Equatorial drusen

Inner Neurosensory Layer

Vitreous Base Excavations

A vitreous base excavation is an ovoid depression involving the inner (vitreal) one-third of neurosensory retina and is located within the anterior half of the peripheral retina (see page 13). Vitreous base excavations have sharp margins without vitreoretinal attachments. The major axis of the oval is usually oriented in a meridional plane. Often there is some pigment dispersion of the retinal pigment epithelium noted at its base and the neurosensory retinal vascular pattern has been reported as normal. There is loss of retinal tissue on its inner (vitreal) surface, yet necrosis, microcystoid degeneration, and glial proliferative elements are absent.

Vitreous base excavations are found in 10% of adults and are bilateral in 43% of cases. In 50% of affected eyes, there is one lesion per eye, and the remaining 50% of affected eyes have from 2 to 7 lesions per eye. Vitreous base excavations have a predilection for the superonasal (horizontal meridian) quadrant. In 18% of meridional folds there is an associated vitreous base excavation, and 20% of meridional complexes have an associated vitreous base excavation. More importantly, vitreous base excavations are rarely associated with retinal holes and retinal detachments.

Retinal Holes

Retinal discontinuities that have no tractional element in their pathogenesis are termed *retinal holes*. These trophic lesions are usually round with smooth edges and do not have an associated retinal flap or vitreous operculum. More specifically, abnormal vitreoretinal attachments are absent. There is minimal reactive gliosis, with a localized degeneration of all retinal elements. There is no overt disturbance in the overlying vitreous, with only minimally reactive retinal pigment epithelium changes subjacent to the retinal hole site.

The incidence of retinal holes is 0.2 to 0.4% of adult eyes, yet some autopsy data suggest a higher incidence. Retinal holes tend to be unilateral, and there is no specific quadrant predilection. About 70% of retinal holes are located within the anterior zone of the peripheral retina (see page 13). Anterior zone retinal holes are rarely associated with retinal detachments, whereas posterior zone retinal holes are more commonly associated with retinal detachments.

Trophic Retinal Degenerations   **Plate 16**

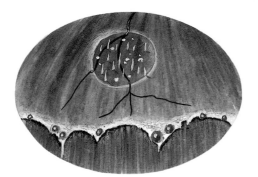

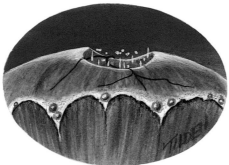

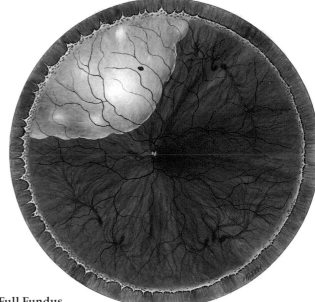

**Vitreous Base Excavations
with Scleral Depression**

Trophic Retinal Holes with Retinal Detachment — Full Fundus

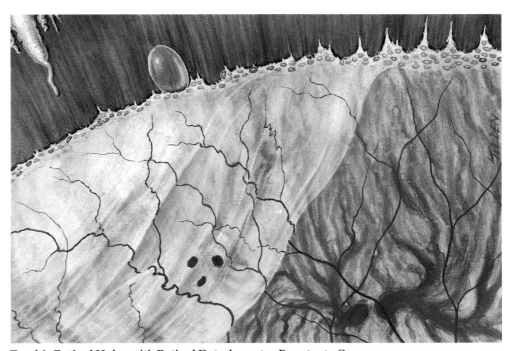

Trophic Retinal Holes with Retinal Detachment — Equator to Ora

Middle Neurosensory Layer

Typical Cystoid Degeneration

Typical cystoid degeneration is the most common peripheral degeneration of the retina characterized by the development of Blessig-Iwanoff cystic spaces in the middle layers (outer plexiform and inner nuclear) of the neurosensory retina. The cystic spaces coalesce to form a labyrinth of tunnels separated by pillars of Müller (glial) cells. On occasion, the inner walls may rupture, giving way to retinal excavations that are unrelated to vitreous base excavations. This cystoid excavation can be mistaken for a retinal hole, but it is usually not a complete hole because there is still some intact retinal tissue at its base. Retinal detachments rarely occur around these pseudoretinal holes. The remaining Müller cells are responsible for the stippled appearance of the inner retinal surface in typical cystoid degeneration.

Typical cystoid degeneration usually begins at the base of a dentate process, at the ora serrata, and advances posteriorly and then circumferentially. The average size of a cystoid lesion is 0.15 mm in diameter. Anterior patches of cystoid degeneration tend to have a larger lesion unit size than posterior patches. The overall shape of a zone of typical cystoid degeneration is parabaloid in the temporal quadrants, whereas in the nasal quadrants it can be parabaloid, club-shaped, or fan-shaped. In exceptional cases, typical cystoid degeneration can extend as far as 13 mm posterior to the ora serrata. Cystoid degeneration can progress posteriorly around paving-stone degeneration, but the following lesions act as barriers to advancing typical cystoid degeneration:

  Lattice retinal degeneration
  Retinal holes
  Chorioretinal scars
  Large retinal vessels

The incidence of typical cystoid degeneration is 100 % of eyes in individuals twenty years and older. It increases in severity with age, leveling off at the seventh decade. There is no specific sexual predilection up to the age of forty years. After forty years, females show more advanced stages of cystoid degeneration than males. There is bilateral mirror symmetry between eyes and there is a predilection for the superior and temporal quadrants.

Typical cystoid degeneration is related to acquired typical degenerative retinoschisis, but it is not related to the following conditions:

  Globe size
    Axial (anteroposterior) length
    Cross-sectional (equatorial) diameter
  Gross features of the vitreous body
  Chorioretinal lesions
  Lattice retinal degeneration
  Paving-stone degeneration
  Pars plana cysts

The relationship of typical cystoid degeneration to retinal tear formation and development of retinal detachments is not known. However, in one study of retinal tears reported in the literature, 61 % had an operculum, and 9 % of those cases had cystoid degeneration. The remaining retinal tears (39 %) did not have an operculum, and of those 14 % had cystoid degeneration in and around the tear site. Very few retinal breaks result from ruptured cystoid spaces in cystoid degeneration, and still fewer develop retinal detachments.

Typical Cystoid Degeneration **Plate 17**

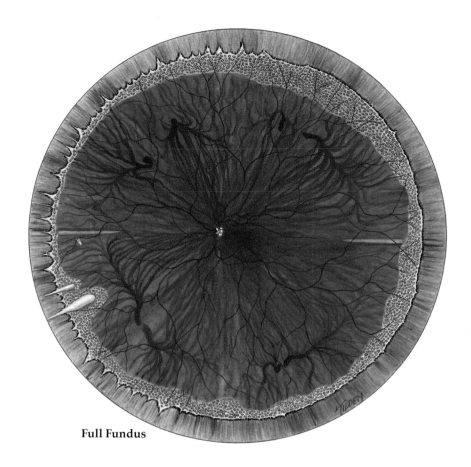

Full Fundus

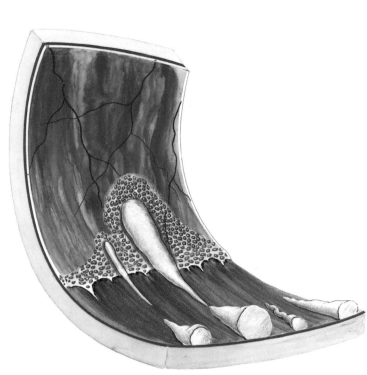

Meridional Complex with Typical Cystoid Degeneration

Ora Serrata Region

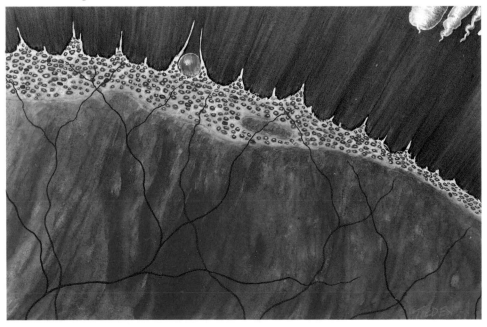

Plate 18   **Reticular Cystoid Degeneration**

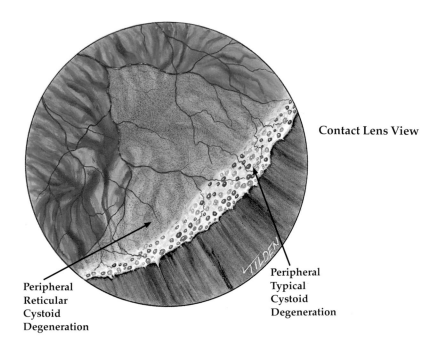

Contact Lens View

Peripheral
Reticular
Cystoid
Degeneration

Peripheral
Typical
Cystoid
Degeneration

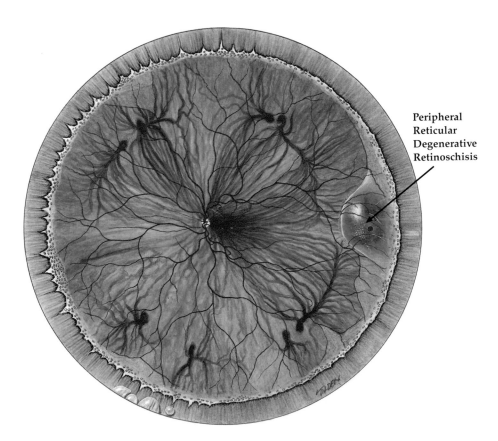

Peripheral
Reticular
Degenerative
Retinoschisis

Reticular Cystoid Degeneration

Reticular cystoid degeneration is a second type of cystoid degeneration in the peripheral retina characterized by cystic spaces bounded by the inner plexiform layer and the internal limiting membrane. Reticular cystoid degeneration has a finely stippled appearance (delicate retinal pillars) and is best detected with contact lens biomicroscopy. Typically it is located posterior to and continuous with an existing patch of typical cystoid degeneration. Reticular cystoid degeneration is often delimited posteriorly by large retinal vessels, which give patches of it its overall linear, rectangular, or trapezoidal shape.

Reticular cystoid degeneration is present in 18.1% of adults or 12.9% of adult eyes with a peak incidence in the fourth through the seventh decades. There is no particular sexual preference, and it is bilateral in 41.4% of patients. There is a predilection for the inferotemporal quadrant. In some individuals, reticular cystoid degeneration may be the precursor lesion of reticular degenerative retinoschisis.

Acquired Typical Degenerative Retinoschisis

Typical degenerative retinoschisis consists of a split in the neurosensory retina, usually at the outer plexiform layer, that is greater than one disc diameter in area. Characteristically, there is tissue loss in the middle layers of the neurosensory retina with disruption of Müller cells (radial pillars), resulting in a round or oval lesion in which the inner portion of the retina is elevated and has a smooth dome-shaped appearance. The retinoschisis cavity is usually optically empty and filled with a clear fluid containing hyaluronic acid. The retinoschisis cavity is surrounded by typical cystoid degeneration. The retinal vessels are located on the retinal dome and are often sheathed. Snowflake lesions are also present on the dome's ceiling surface (facing the retinoschisis cavity) and represent the ends of broken Müller fibers. The dome itself is fairly rigid, and it does not move or undulate with movements of the globe, as do retina bullae in the typical rhegmatogenous retinal detachment. Also, the appearance of the retinoschisis dome does not change relative to gravity, as do the retinal bullae (shifting fluid) of an exudative retinal detachment. The outer layer of the retinoschisis lesion often is of irregular thickness, but usually is attached to the retinal pigment epithelium. Retinoschisis lesions cut the vertical transmission lines of the photoreceptor cells to the ganglion cells, resulting in absolute visual field cuts. Most patients are totally unaware of their visual deficits because of the gradual onset of the lesions.

Typical degenerative retinoschisis is found in 3.5% of adults and is bilateral in 33% to 82% of these individuals, with a predilection for the inferotemporal quadrant (72%).

Twenty-eight percent of retinoschisis lesions are found in the superotemporal quadrant. The peak incidence is in the fifth decade. Retinal holes are extremely infrequent in either the inner and/or outer layers, as is the incidence of retinal detachments. Treatment of retinal breaks in typical degenerative retinoschisis is rarely indicated. Also, posterior extension of the retinoschisis process to the macular region does not as a rule occur in typical degenerative retinoschisis. Hyperopia is the most common refractive error associated with retinoschisis.

Reticular Degenerative Retinoschisis

A second form of retinoschisis is reticular degenerative retinoschisis, which is characterized by more tissue destruction than is found in typical degenerative retinoschisis. Reticular degenerative retinoschisis consists of a round or ovoid bullous elevation of extremely thin neurosensory retina (inner layer) containing retinal blood vessels and is located in the retinal periphery. The posterior border of the retinoschisis cavity often extends to the equator. Reticular cystoid degeneration is usually found at the edges of the retinoschisis cavity, and typical cystoid degeneration (100%) is usually found anterior to the schisis cavity at the ora serrata region.

Sclerosis or sheathing of retinal vessels is often present on the dome of the retinoschisis lesion, and there is an optically empty cavity presumably containing hyaluronic acid material. The outer wall of the retina often has a honeycomb appearance due to irregular excavations and atrophy of the retinal tissue. Snowflakes representing broken ends of Müller fibers are also present on the ceiling surface (facing the schisis cavity) of the dome. The major tissue loss is seen in the inner layers of the retina, especially at the nerve fiber layer, in contrast to typical degenerative retinoschisis, where the splitting and major tissue loss is at the outer plexiform layer.

Reticular degenerative retinoschisis is found in 1.6% of adults and is bilateral in 15% of these individuals. There is a peak incidence in the fourth through seventh decades, and there is no particular sexual predilection in that males and females appear to be equally affected. There is a predilection for the inferotemporal quadrant, and 7% of cases have an associated macular degeneration.

In reticular degenerative retinoschisis, the incidence of outer layer breaks is 25%, and the incidence of inner layer breaks is 16%. The incidence of retinal detachments is 22%. Of those reticular degenerative retinoschisis patients who present with a retinal detachment, 77% had retinal breaks in both inner and outer layers and 16% had outer layer breaks alone.

Acquired Typical and Reticular Degenerative Retinoschisis   **Plate 19**

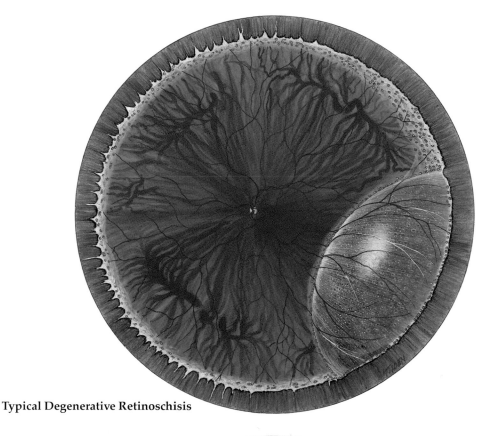

Typical Degenerative Retinoschisis

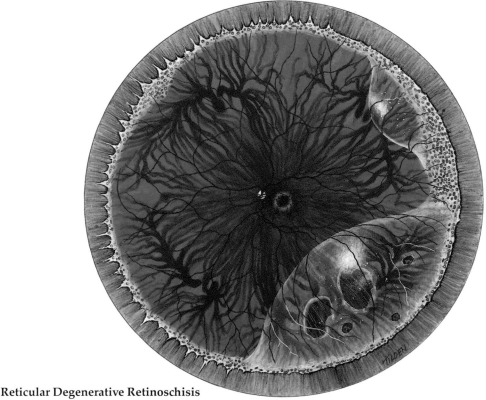

Reticular Degenerative Retinoschisis

Outer Neurosensory Layer – Retinal Pigment Epithelium

Paving-Stone (Cobblestone) Degeneration

Characteristically, paving-stone or cobblestone degeneration consists of discrete yellow-white chorioretinal lesions (0.1 to 1.5 mm in diameter) between the equator and the ora serrata. There is a loss of pigment in the retinal pigment epithelium often allowing visibility of subjacent choroidal vessels. Also, there is atrophy of the outer portion of the overlying neurosensory retina, including photoreceptor cells and the external limiting membrane. Presumably, paving-stone degeneration is due to shutdown of a zone of choriocapillaris vessels and the overlying neurosensory retina is adherent to remnants of the retinal pigment epithelium and Bruch's membrane. Paving-stone degeneration lesions may be single round lesions, or they may coalesce, forming scalloped borders, often with hyperpigmented edges due to pigment migration from the centers of the lesions.

Paving-stone degeneration lesions do not have abnormal vitreoretinal adhesions and are present in 22 to 27% of adults over 20 years of age with a peak incidence in the fifth through the seventh decades. The incidence of paving-stone degeneration does increase with age and is bilateral in 38% of affected individuals. Of the bilateral cases, 75% have symmetrical (mirror image) lesions. There is no particular sexual predilection: males and females are equally affected. Paving-stone degeneration lesions have a predilection for the inferotemporal quadrant, usually sparing the horizontal meridians.

Paving-stone degeneration rarely leads to retinal breaks and retinal detachments, therefore its presence does not warrant prophylactic treatment. However, cases have been observed where retinal detachment traction forces have secondarily created a retinal break at a paving-stone degeneration lesion site and under these circumstances the breaks should be treated.

Peripheral Tapetochoroidal (Honeycomb) Degeneration

Peripheral tapetochoroidal or honeycomb degeneration is a pigmentary disturbance of the retinal pigment epithelium appearing as a circumferential band at the equator in elderly individuals. There is irregularity in the pigment, consisting of increased granularity in the form of irregular hyperpigmented lines in a honeycomb or reticular arrangement. In addition, there is also diffuse depigmentation of the retinal pigment epithelium between the equator and ora serrata. Underneath the vitreous base there is less pigment loss in the retinal pigment epithelium than at the equator.

Histologically, there is diminution of the choriocapillaris, diffuse thickening of Bruch's membrane, loss of melanin granules from the retinal pigment epithelium, and loss of some of the photoreceptor cells.

The incidence of peripheral tapetochoroidal (honeycomb) degeneration is approximately 20% of adults over the age of 40 years and is invariably bilateral in 100% of affected cases. There may be an associated visual field constriction in this age-related condition. Peripheral tapetochoroidal degeneration does not lead to retinal breaks or retinal detachments and does not require specific treatment.

Equatorial Drusen

Equatorial drusen consist of yellow-white colloid bodies of the retinal pigment epithelium and are more common than drusen of the macula. Equatorial drusen are more common in the aged and are often found nasally, in association with senile tapetochoroidal (honeycomb) pigmentary degeneration. The drusen can occur singly, in clusters, or in a geographic pattern, and they do not appear to be related specifically to macular drusen and senile macular degeneration. Equatorial drusen may be limited to one quadrant or, more frequently, distributed among serveral quadrants. On rare occasions, subretinal neovascularization, hemorrhage, and subretinal fluid can develop from equatorial drusen.

From a physiologic point of view, patients with equatorial drusen usually have normal visual fields and electroretinograms. However, the electrooculogram and dark adaptation tests may be either normal or slightly reduced.

The origin of drusen is still debated, but most likely it represents incompletely digested remnants of outer segments of photoreceptor cells in aging retinal pigment epithelial cells that have not been cleared away by the choriocapillaris system. In some cases, drusen have an autosomal dominant hereditary transmission.

Paving-Stone Degeneration, Honeycomb Degeneration, and Equatorial Drusen　　**Plate 20**

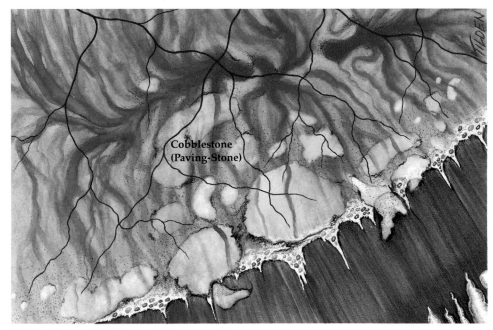

Paving-Stone (Cobblestone) Degeneration

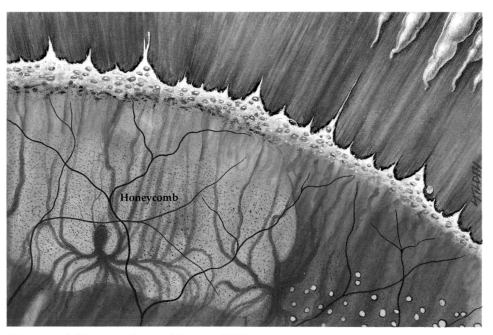

Honeycomb Degeneration and Equatorial Drusen

Tractional Retinal Degenerations 5

Anatomic Classification of Retinal Tears

Oral tears occur at the ora serrata, whereas *intrabasal tears* are located within the vitreous base. *Juxtabasal tears* are located at the posterior border of the vitreous base. *Extrabasal tears* are located within the region bounded by the equator and posterior border of the vitreous base. Retinal tears can be partial thickness involving the inner (vitreal) portion of the neurosensory retina or they can be through and through, in which case they are termed full-thickness retinal tears (see Table 5.1).

Partial-Thickness Peripheral Retinal Tears

Intrabasal Partial-Thickness Tears
Partial-thickness retinal tears may be operculated or have a U- or V-shaped retinal flap. This type of tear may be related to a zonular traction tuft or perhaps a noncystic retinal tuft.

Juxtabasal Partial-Thickness Tears
Juxtabasal partial-thickness retinal tears are found in 12% of adults, and 5% of affected cases are bilateral. These partial-thickness tears usually develop as a result of a posterior vitreous detachment. There is no particular quadrant predilection.

Extrabasal Partial-Thickness Tears
Extrabasal partial-thickness tears occur posterior to the vitreous base and often are related to avulsion of a paravascular vitreoretinal attachment during an active posterior cortical vitreous detachment. In other instances, partial-thickness extrabasal tears are due to an avulsion of a cystic retinal tuft with or without an associated posterior vitreous detachment.

Paravascular partial-thickness extrabasal tears occur in 17% of adults and are bilateral in 27% of cases with a predilection for the superior peripheral quadrants. These tears usually do not, in and of themselves, cause a retinal detachment, but may lead to retinal and vitreous hemorrhages. However, it is important to note that there is an association of full-thickness tears with the presence of partial-thickness peripheral retinal tears!

Table 5.1.
Tractional Retinal Degenerations
Partial-thickness retinal tears
Oral
Intrabasal
Juxtabasal
Extrabasal
Full-thickness retinal tears
Oral
Dialyses (juvenile)
Avulsion of vitreous base
Giant retinal tears
Intrabasal
Juxtabasal
Extrabasal

Full-Thickness Peripheral Retinal Tears

Full-thickness retinal tears consist of a complete through and through break or discontinuity in the neurosensory retina and have an associated retinal flap or overlying vitreous operculum. With aging, there is shrinkage of the operculum or retinal flap and mottling of the subjacent retinal pigment epithelium is seen. In general, full-thickness retinal tears have abnormal vitreoretinal tractional forces that participate in the formation of the tear. The overall incidence of all full-thickness retinal tears is 4.4% of adults and is bilateral in 11% of affected cases, with a predilection for the inferior and temporal quadrants. Of all full-thickness peripheral retinal tears, the incidence of retinal flaps is 39% and the incidence of opercula is 61%.

Histologic observations of the retinal tear flap show tissue shrinkage, glial proliferation, retinal degeneration, cystoid degeneration, and abnormal vitreoretinal attachments. The margins of retinal tears reveal significant amounts of retinal arteriosclerosis. In the region of the retinal tear, choroidal sclerosis as well as degeneration and, on occasion, hyperplasia of the retinal pigment epithelium are found.

Anatomic Classification of Retinal Tears   Plate 21

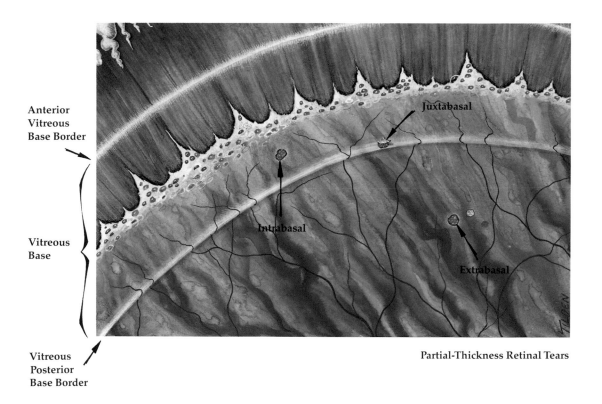

Anterior
Vitreous
Base Border

Vitreous
Base

Vitreous
Posterior
Base Border

Juxtabasal

Intrabasal

Extrabasal

Partial-Thickness Retinal Tears

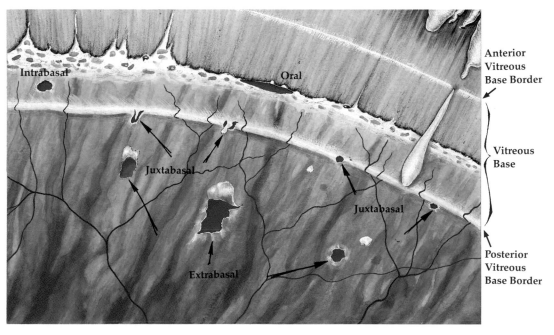

Intrabasal

Oral

Juxtabasal

Juxtabasal

Extrabasal

Anterior
Vitreous
Base Border

Vitreous
Base

Posterior
Vitreous
Base Border

Full-Thickness Retinal Tears

Oral Full-Thickness Tears

Oral full-thickness tears result from posterior movement of the vitreous base and are located at the ora serrata. Most other peripheral retinal tears occur as a result of anterior movement of the vitreous base. In full-thickness oral tears, tractional forces are vectored posteriorly, and in some cases there is a complete avulsion of a portion of the vitreous base. This can occur in cases of developmental anomalies or from trauma. Avulsion of the vitreous base in the inferotemporal or superonasal quadrant is believed to be pathognomonic of antecedent trauma to the eye. However, a number of superonasal and inferotemporal oral tears are unrelated to trauma.

A large full-thickness oral tear is termed a *retinal dialysis* and may eventually form a retinal detachment. If the tear is greater than 3 clock hours or 90° in circumference, it is termed a *giant retinal tear.*

Because oral tears are often associated with antecedent ocular trauma, they tend to occur in younger individuals and more commonly in males than females. The peak age of incidence is 20 years, and this condition is rarely seen after the fifth decade.

Retinal Dialyses (Juvenile)

Retinal dialyses are oral tears at the posterior edge of the ora serrata with almost no tendency of the tear flap to form posterior rolled edges. Often there are subretinal demarcation lines that are white or black-brown, concentric with the retinal tear.

Some cases of retinal dialyses are due to trauma, others are spontaneous and may be genetic in origin. Spontaneous retinal dialyses are often asymptomatic and bilateral, occurring preferentially in the inferotemporal quadrant in young individuals. There is no sexual predilection: males and females are equally affected. The progression of the retinal detachment is insidious, and patients usually do not complain of visual loss until the macular region detaches.

Avulsion of the Vitreous Base

The vitreous base is firmly attached to the peripheral neurosensory retina as well as to the nonpigmented epithelium of the pars plana. In cases of substantial blunt trauma to the globe, avulsion of the vitreous base can take place most commonly in the superonasal quadrant. Ophthalmoscopically, one sees a strip of nonpigmented epithelium dangling like a rope in the vitreous cavity overlying the peripheral retina, which is usually torn as well. There may be an associated retinal detachment. A disinserted or dangling vitreous base is usually prima facie evidence of previous ocular trauma to the eye.

Retinal Dialyses **Plate 22**

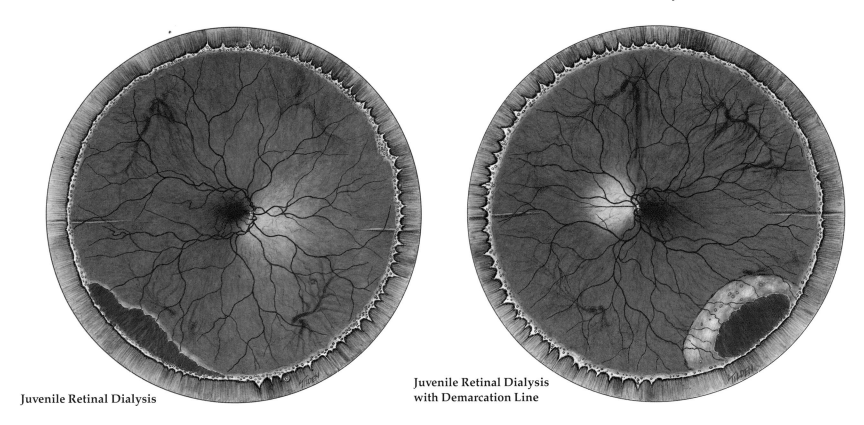

Juvenile Retinal Dialysis

Juvenile Retinal Dialysis
with Demarcation Line

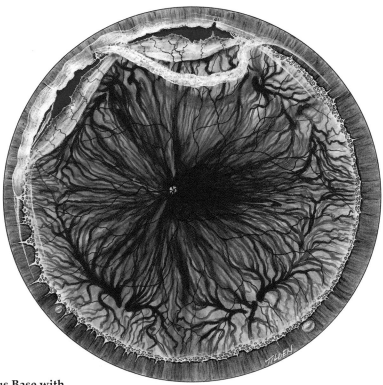

Avulsion of Vitreous Base with
Retinal Dialysis and Early Retinal Detachment

Giant Retinal Tears

Giant retinal tears are tears greater than 90° in circumferential length and may be spontaneous or due to trauma (20%). Thirty percent of cases occur in aphakic eyes. High myopes with lattice degeneration are especially at risk. Spontaneous cases, usually in males, occur without any warning. Twenty percent of cases have a familial history of retinal detachment. On occasion, giant retinal tears have been seen with colobomas of the lens-zonule system.

Giant retinal tears occur near the ora serrata, and usually there is a thin zone of elevated retina remaining attached at the ora serrata. There is a tendency for the giant tear flap to roll posteriorly and scroll up, in contrast to a retinal dialysis flap, which does not tend to fold posteriorly. The surgical and visual prognosis is extremely poor in giant retinal tears, whereas it is quite good in retinal dialyses. There is a high percentage of bilaterality in giant retinal tears.

Intrabasal Full-Thickness Retinal Tears

Intrabasal full-thickness retinal tears are located within the vitreous base and usually result from either a subtotal or complete avulsion of a preexisting retinal zonular traction tuft. There is no relationship of these tears to tractional forces acting along the posterior border of the vitreous base or to those forces created by a posterior cortical vitreous detachment. In addition, these tears do not appear to be related to advancing age, lattice degeneration, or trauma. Intrabasal full-thickness tears are rare and infrequently lead to retinal detachment.

Juxtabasal Full-Thickness Retinal Tears

Juxtabasal full-thickness retinal tears are invariably due to asymmetric tractional forces distributed along the posterior border of the vitreous base during an active posterior cortical vitreous detachment. These tears are almost always associated with a retinal flap and are the most common of the full-thickness retinal tears and carry the highest risk of developing a retinal detachment. Developmental variations and lattice retinal degeneration lesions create irregularities at the posterior border of the vitreous base and are therefore predisposing lesions for the development of juxtabasal full-thickness tears during a posterior cortical vitreous detachment. These lesions allow unequal distribution of tractional forces during the vitreous detachment process.

Extrabasal Full-Thickness Retinal Tears

Avulsions of cystic retinal tufts are often associated with a free vitreous operculum and represent the classic *extrabasal full-thickness retinal tear* which usually occurs in association with a posterior cortical vitreous detachment. These tears are not as common as the juxtabasal full-thickness retinal tears. On occasion, equatorial lattice retinal degeneration lesions may, in the presence of a posterior vitreous detachment, lead to the formation of an extrabasal full-thickness retinal tear. Pure extrabasal full-thickness operculated retinal tears do not, as a rule, produce total retinal detachments, but can lead to a localized retinal detachment usually one to two disc diameters in size.

Full-Thickness Peripheral Retinal Tears **Plate 23**

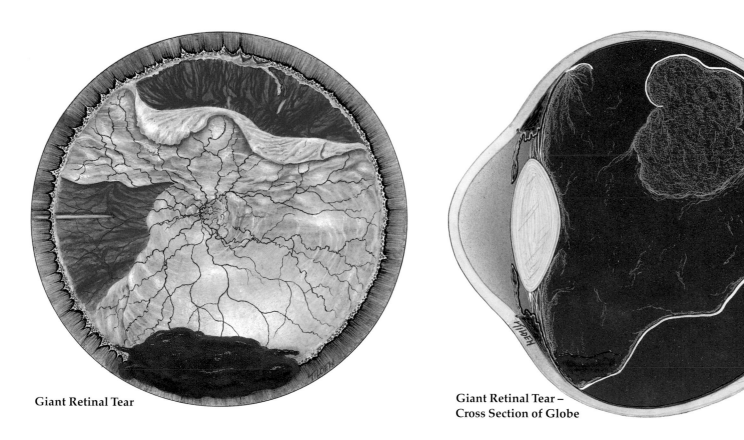

Giant Retinal Tear

**Giant Retinal Tear –
Cross Section of Globe**

Full Thickness Retinal Tears

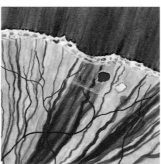

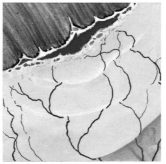

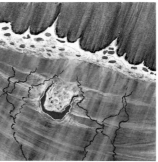

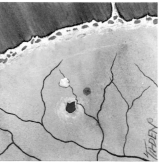

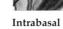

Oral Intrabasal Juxtabasal Extrabasal

Trophic and Tractional Retinal Degenerations

6

The disorders in this section have trophic (nutritional and/or vascular) and tractional components that play a major role in their pathogenesis (see Table 6.1).

Table 6.1. Trophic and Tractional Retinal Degenerations
White-without-pressure
White-with-pressure
Snail-track degeneration
Lattice retinal degeneration

Hereditary vitreoretinal degenerations
    Wagner's hereditary vitreoretinal degeneration
    Stickler's syndrome
    Congenital hereditary retinoschisis (juvenile)
    Goldmann-Favre disease
    Familial exudative vitreoretinopathy
    Snowflake degeneration

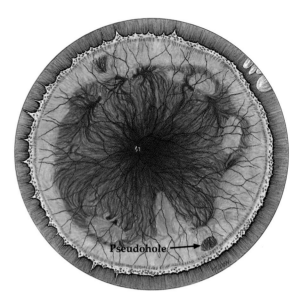

Geographic, White-without-Pressure

White-with- or -without-Pressure

White-without-Pressure
Normally the peripheral fundus is transparent when viewed with an indirect ophthalmoscope. When scleral depression is applied, there is no change in the transparency of the retina in the region of the scleral depression. However, in some individuals the retina appears translucent as a result of the scleral depression, and this has been termed white-with-pressure.

White-without-pressure refers to areas of peripheral retina that have a whitish translucent watered-silk appearance without scleral depression. The etiology of this condition remains obscure but may be related to vitreous traction. White-without-pressure is found more frequently in myopes and in dark-skinned people, for example, Negroes and people from the Mediterranean region. Often there are sharply demarcated edges to these geographic-shaped lesions. The lesions are usually located between the ora serrata and the equator. Often white-without-pressure lesions can be found posterior to the equator.

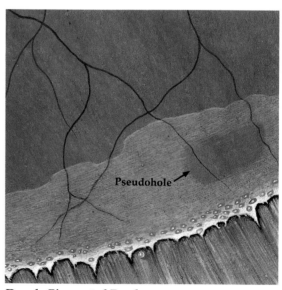

**Deeply Pigmented Fundus,
White-without-Pressure, Pseudohole**

Histopathology findings in regions of white-without-pressure include localized vitreoretinal adhesions, retinal atrophy of nuclear layers, cystoid degeneration, hyalinization of retinal arterioles, vitreous syneresis cavities, and posterior vitreous detachments. There does not appear to be any association of white-without-pressure lesions with retinal holes, tears, or retinal detachments.

White-with-Pressure
White-with-pressure is a whitish translucent bandlike lesion of the peripheral retinal usually located between the ora serrata and the equator. When the scleral depressor is applied to the outer surface of the globe, there is an indentation of the wall of the eye, and the retina goes from a transparent state to an opalescent state with some obscuration of the subjacent retinal pigment epithelium and choroidal vasculature. The borders of white-with-pressure have complex contours (geographic) and on occasion may even partially or completely surround a small region of normal retina which may be mistaken for a retinal hole, but it is really a pseudoretinal hole.

White-with-pressure should be differentiated from a flat

White-with- or without-Pressure   **Plate 24**

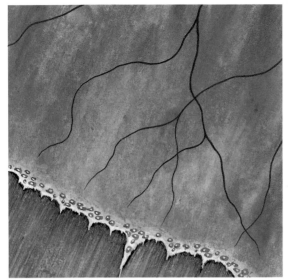

Normal Peripheral Fundus (no Scleral Depression)

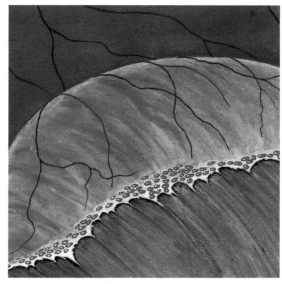

Normal Fundus with Scleral Depression

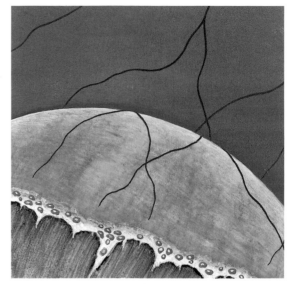

White-with-Pressure with Scleral Depression

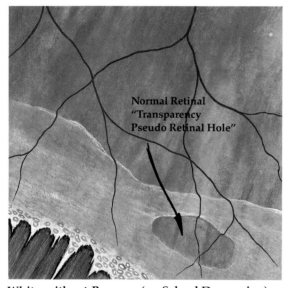

White-without-Pressure (no Scleral Depression)

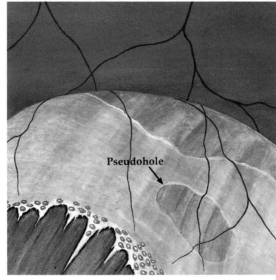

White-with-Pressure with Scleral Depression

or shallow retinal detachment, extensive cystoid degeneration, and flat degenerative retinoschisis lesions. White-with-pressure is also often seen at the edges of lattice retinal degeneration and cystoid degeneration.

The origin of white-with-pressure is still not well established, but may represent a weakness in the extracellular substance located in the subretinal space between the retinal pigment epithelium and the outer segments of the photoreceptor cells.

The incidence of white-with-pressure is over 30% of adult eyes and most cases are bilateral. Only 5% of people under 20 years of age have white-with-pressure, whereas 66% of those over 70 years of age have white-with-pressure. There is increased incidence of white-with-pressure with increased myopia, and the incidence approaches 100% in eyes with an anteroposterior or axial length of 33 mm or greater. It is more common in darkly pigmented fundi. Males are equally affected with this condition as are females. There is a predilection for the peripheral retina in the temporal quadrants and white-with-pressure lesions do not appear to be associated with retinal breaks.

Snail-Track Retinal Degeneration

Snail-track degeneration has been described as a variation or early stage of lattice retinal degeneration by some authors, while others have felt that it is a closely related, yet separate entity. Snail-track degeneration, or *"Schneckenspuren"* as Gonin termed it, consists of sharply demarcated bands of thin neurosensory retinal tissue, which have a crinkled or frosted appearance on their inner surface.

Characteristically, white vessel or lattice changes as well as retinal pigment abnormalities (deposits) are absent in snail-track degeneration, in contrast to lattice retinal degeneration. Retinal holes without opercula are found in snail-track degeneration in the following quadrantic distribution: inferotemporal quadrant 54%, superotemporal quadrant 18%, superonasal quadrant 16% and the inferonasal quadrant 12%. There is syneresis of the vitreous gel in affected eyes in 100% of cases and the incidence of retinal detachments in these eyes has been reported as high as 48%.

In these cases, 80% of the snail-track lesions are located within the anterior half of the peripheral retina; 90% are in myopic eyes, with 33% in highly myopic eyes. Snail-track degeneration lesions have a predilection for the superonasal and superotemporal quadrants. There is an autosomal recessive transmission tendency, and males and females are equally affected.

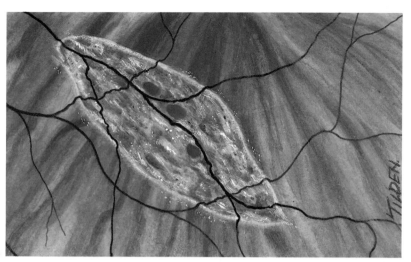

Snail-Track Degeneration – Fundus

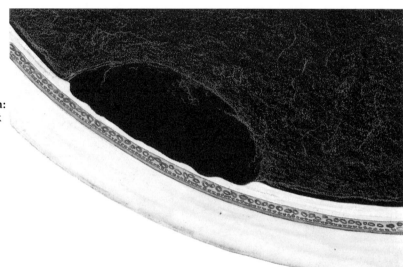

Snail-Track Degeneration – Cross Section:
Liquefaction of Vitreous over Snail-Track
Lesion

Lattice Retinal Degeneration

Gonin was the first to describe *Schneckenspuren* in 1904, which was later renamed lattice retinal degeneration in the 1950s. *Lattice retinal degeneration* consists of a sharply demarcated circumferentially oriented lesion characterized by thinning of the inner portion (vitreal) of the neurosensory retina, white lines, and a pigmentary disturbance. There is an arborizing network of "sheathed" retinal vessels due to an obliterative fibrosis reaction, which is seen ophthalmoscopically as a series of white lines crisscrossing one another. Schepens coined the term "lattice" to describe this network of white blood vessels within the lesion site. Lattice retinal vessels are present in about 46% of cases. In 92% of the cases a pigmentary disturbance is found in the subjacent retinal pigment epithelium, consisting of depigmentation zones and clumps of hyperpigmentation as well as perivascular pigmentation of neurosensory retina within the lattice degeneration lesion.

There is a focal thinning of the inner portion of the retina with loss of retinal neurons and thinning of the internal limiting membrane. Sometimes there are areas where the internal limiting membrane is absent, and glial cells manufacture additional internal limiting (basement) membrane, which is seen ophthalmoscopically as greyish-white particles on the inner surface of the lattice lesions. Invariably, there is liquefaction of the vitreous over the lattice lesions with abnormal vitreoretinal attachments at the margins of the lattice lesions. Retinal tear sites, when they develop, tend to do so along the margins of the lattice degeneration lesion.

Most lattice lesions are found anterior to the equator and two thirds of them are in the vertical meridians between the 11 o'clock and 1 o'clock meridians superiorly and between the 5 o'clock and 7 o'clock meridians inferiorly. The major axis of the lattice lesion is oriented parallel to the equator and is termed *equatorial lattice degeneration* (68%). Radial (7%) or paravascular lattice degeneration (parallels retinal vessels) is less common than the equatorial type and is located more posteriorly. There is focal thinning (19.2%) of the inner portion of the neurosensory retina and round or oval retinal holes are noted in 18.2 to 31.0% of cases. Retinal tears are found in 1.4% of eyes with lattice degeneration, and for the most part these are situated at the lateral or posterior edges of the lattice lesion.

Of all retinal detachments, lattice degeneration lesions are present in 41% of cases, and it is thought that lattice degeneration is the major cause of the detachment process in 21% of cases. In 55 to 70% of these cases, a tear developing at the posterior or lateral border of the lattice lesion is responsible for the detachment, whereas in 30 to 45% of cases atrophic holes within the lattice lesion are responsible for the development of the retinal detachment. Most of the patients who develop retinal detachments due to lattice degeneration are over 50 years of age, and 43% of these eyes are myopic.

The overall incidence of lattice degeneration is from 6 to 7.9% of the adult population, with males and females equally affected. The onset is usually in the second decade of life and tends to be bilateral in 33 to 50% of cases. Lattice degeneration is more common in myopic eyes than in hyperopic eyes. The incidence of lattice retinal degeneration increases with increasing axial length of the globe. There is usually no hereditary pattern in lattice retinal degeneration; however, in some families an autosomal dominant transmission has been mapped out.

Lattice Retinal Degeneration   **Plate 26**

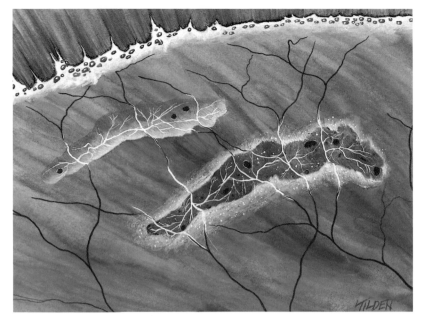

Lattice Retinal Degeneration with Atrophic Holes

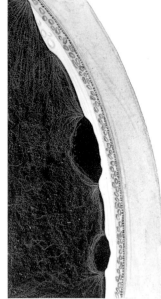

**Lattice Retinal Degeneration – Cross Section:
Liquified Vitreous over Lattice Lesions**

**Lattice Degeneration with Horseshoe Tears
and Localized Retinal Detachment**

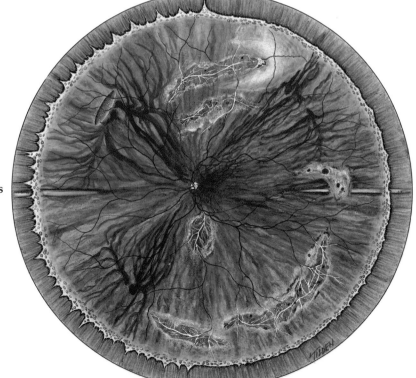

Plate 27   **Wagner's Hereditary Vitreoretinal Degeneration**

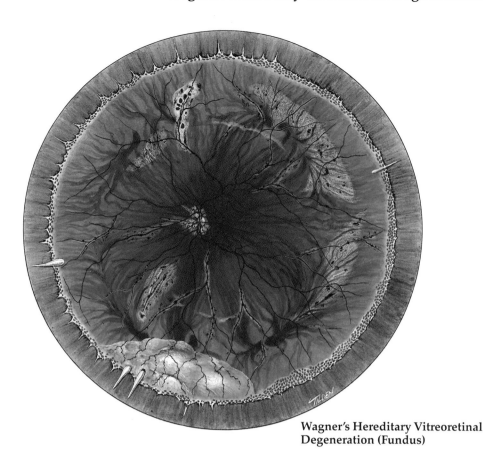

Wagner's Hereditary Vitreoretinal
Degeneration (Fundus)

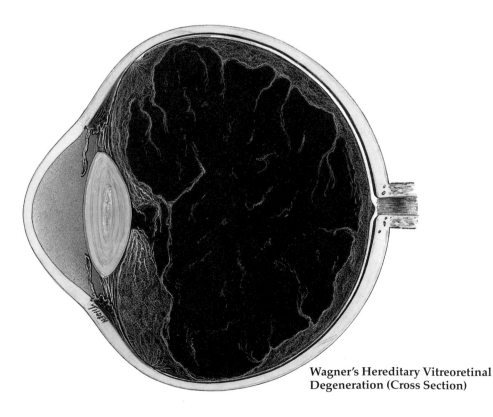

Wagner's Hereditary Vitreoretinal
Degeneration (Cross Section)

Hereditary Vitreoretinal Degenerations

Hereditary vitreoretinal degenerations consist of a group of disorders primarily affecting the vitreous and retina with a distinct hereditary pattern and are listed in Table 6.1. Systemic disorders associated with some of the vitreoretinal degenerations are enumerated in Table 6.2.

Table 6.1. Hereditary Vitreoretinal Degenerations
Wagner's hereditary vitreoretinal degeneration
Stickler's syndrome
Congenital hereditary retinoschisis (juvenile)
Goldmann-Favre's disease
Familial exudative vitreoretinopathy
Snowflake degeneration

Table 6.2. Systemic Conditions Associated with Vitreoretinal Degenerations
Marfan's syndrome
Homocystinuria
Ehlers-Danlos syndrome
Pseudoxanthoma elasticum

Wagner's Hereditary Vitreoretinal Degeneration

Wagner first described this hereditary vitreoretinal degeneration in 1938. Characteristically, there is a large syneresis cavity behind the lens with membranous condensations of the vitreous body (bands and veils). There is a high incidence of cataracts and retinal detachment in this autosomal dominant disease, which is usually bilateral. Retinal vessels are narrowed and sheathed with paravascular pigmentation, and there is retinal pigment epithelium atrophy, choroidal atrophy, and, in some cases, optic atrophy. The electroretinogram is understandably subnormal. There is often radial and equatorial lattice degeneration, peripheral degenerative retinoschisis, myopia, and glaucoma found in the eyes of patients with Wagner's hereditary vitreoretinal degeneration (see Table 6.3).

Stickler's Syndrome

In 1965, Stickler described a hereditary progressive arthroophthalmopathy, with associated cleft palate, high myopia (-16 diopters), an optically empty vitreous cavity with fundus pigmentary abnormalities, preretinal membranes, cataracts, and a malignant form of retinal detachment that had an autosomal dominant inheritance pattern. Other systemic findings that have been attributed to Stickler's syndrome include flattened facies, skeletal dysplasia, and, on rare occasions, mental retardation.

The major ophthalmic and systemic abnormalities of Wagner's hereditary vitreoretinal degeneration and Stickler's syndrome are outlined in Table 6.3.

There is a high incidence of retinal detachments in patients with Wagner's disease and/or Stickler's syndrome, and they are difficult to repair because of the vitreoretinal membranes, cataracts, large (5% have giant retinal tears) and multiple retinal tears, and an increased tendency to go on to massive periretinal proliferation. Many cases need vitrectomy in addition to scleral buckling surgery to repair the retinal detachment. The surgical success rate in these cases has been reported to be 68%.

Table 6.3.

Wagner's Hereditary Vitreoretinal Degeneration

Ophthalmic findings
  Large syneresis cavities
  Large lacunae (central and posterior vitreous)
  Vitreous veils (membranous condensations)
  Retinal vessels narrowed
  Retinal vessels sheathed
  Paravascular retinal pigmentation (periphery) (61%)
  Choroidal vessel atrophy (40%)
    Hyperpigmentation
    Hypopigmentation
  Tessellated fundus
  Retinal detachment (50%)
  Atypical posterior vitreous detachments
  Retinal breaks (75%)
  Lattice retinal degeneration (26%)
  Retinoschisis
  Cataracts (after adolescence, 60% incidence)
    Posterior capsular (41%)
    Posterior subcapsular (31%)
    Nuclear sclerosis (28%)
    Mature cataract (28%)
  Optic atrophy (4%)
  Contracted visual fields (ring scotoma)
  Subnormal electroretinogram (ERG)
  Night blindness
  Color vision – normal
  Dark adaptation – decreased
  Glaucoma
  Myopia
  Epicanthus
  Extensive white-with-pressure (35%)
  Meridional folds (17%)

Systemic manifestations (Stickler's syndrome)
  Arthropathy
  Cleft palate
  Flat nose
  Genu valgum
  Micrognathia
  Glossoptosis
  Chondrodysplasia

Congenital Hereditary Retinoschisis
(Juvenile Retinoschisis)

Congenital hereditary retinoschisis involves a splitting of the retina at the nerve fiber layer into an inner and outer layer of retina, which results in absolute scotomas in the visual field corresponding to the zones of schisis. Congenital retinoschisis is most frequently observed in the inferotemporal quadrant and can extend to the posterior pole, but does not, as a rule, extend to the ora serrata region.

Vitreous findings in congenital retinoschisis include a larger than usual Cloquet's canal (early cases with infantile canal proportions) and a prominent fibrous condensation of the cortex. In advanced cases, vitreous bands are found crisscrossing the vitreous gel, which shows widespread nonconfluent liquefaction cavities. The vitreous cortex is usually attached to the inner surface of the retinoschisis cavity and is liquefied over the region of a retinal break in the inner layer. Incomplete posterior vitreous detachment with a collapse of the cortex is frequently observed in cases of retinoschisis, showing giant inner layer holes with a history of recurrent vitreous hemorrhage. Vitreous traction on the retinal vessels may lead to a massive vitreous hemorrhage.

Congenital retinoschisis is usually discovered in children and young adults, but has been detected at birth. Most of the patients see floaters and have poor vision with strabismus or nystagmus. Congenital retinoschisis is invariably bilateral and is transmitted as a sex-linked recessive mode of inheritance. In rare cases, it has been found in females as an autosomal recessive disease.

During the first five years of life, there is usually progression (increased volume of retinoschisis, increased numbers of inner and/or outer layer breaks) and then it levels off and is fairly stable by the age of 20. There are periods of regression usually associated with release of vitreous cortical traction on the inner surface of the retina. The ophthalmoscopic features of congenital retinoschisis are outlined as follows:*

Inner layer is extremely thin, elevated with a smooth dome or balloon shape and is immobile. Retinal vessels are often sheathed and are seen on its inner surface. Inner

* Modified from Tolentino FI, Schepens CL, Freeman HM: Vitreoretinal Disorders/Diagnosis and Management. Philadelphia, W.B. Saunders Company, 1976, pp 251, 254.

layer breaks are often multiple, round or oval, and quite variable in size. In some cases the holes are so large that only the vessels and minimal amounts of atrophic retina are left behind. Gliosis and neovascularization of the inner layer have been observed.

Outer layer is often invisible when it is attached and becomes visible with detachment. The outer layer contains strands of Müller's cells and is avascular. Outer layer breaks are oval and have rolled edges.

Optic disc: pseudopapillitis, pseudopapilledema, "dragging of the disc" and optic-disc pallor (atrophy) have been noted in congenital retinoschisis.

Macula shows cystic retinal changes, giving the appearance of a depigmented star on a background of mottled pigment (beaten copper). This may represent an incomplete form of retinoschisis within the macula that results from a peripheral schisis extension into the macula. Less often, there is independent schisis developing in the macula.

Histopathologic analysis reveals that the splitting takes place at the nerve fiber layer of the retina in congenital retinoschisis, as compared to acquired typical degenerative retinoschisis where the split takes place in the outer plexiform layer. The vitreous cortex is adherent to the inner retinal layer of congenital retinoschisis, and the retinoschisis cavity contains an amorphous proteinaceous material. The vitreous cavity is smaller than normal, and the vitreous gel is located anterior to the inner layer of retinoschisis. Fibrous metaplasia of the macular retinal pigment epithelium is often present.

There is no satisfactory form of treatment for congenital retinoschisis that will restore vision lost from the damaged neurosensory retina at the schisis lesion sites. However, if outer layer breaks are present, photocoagulation or cryosurgery may be of some value. If a retinal detachment develops, then scleral buckling surgery and an encircling band are appropriate. The goal of such surgery would be to close all the outer layer breaks.

The differential diagnosis of congenital retinoschisis includes retinal detachment, acquired typical and reticular degenerative retinoschisis, Eales' disease, retinitis pigmentosa, sickle cell retinopathy, retrolental fibroplasia (cicatricial stage), and persistent hyperplastic primary vitreous.

Congenital Hereditary Retinoschisis **Plate 28**
(Juvenile Retinoschisis)

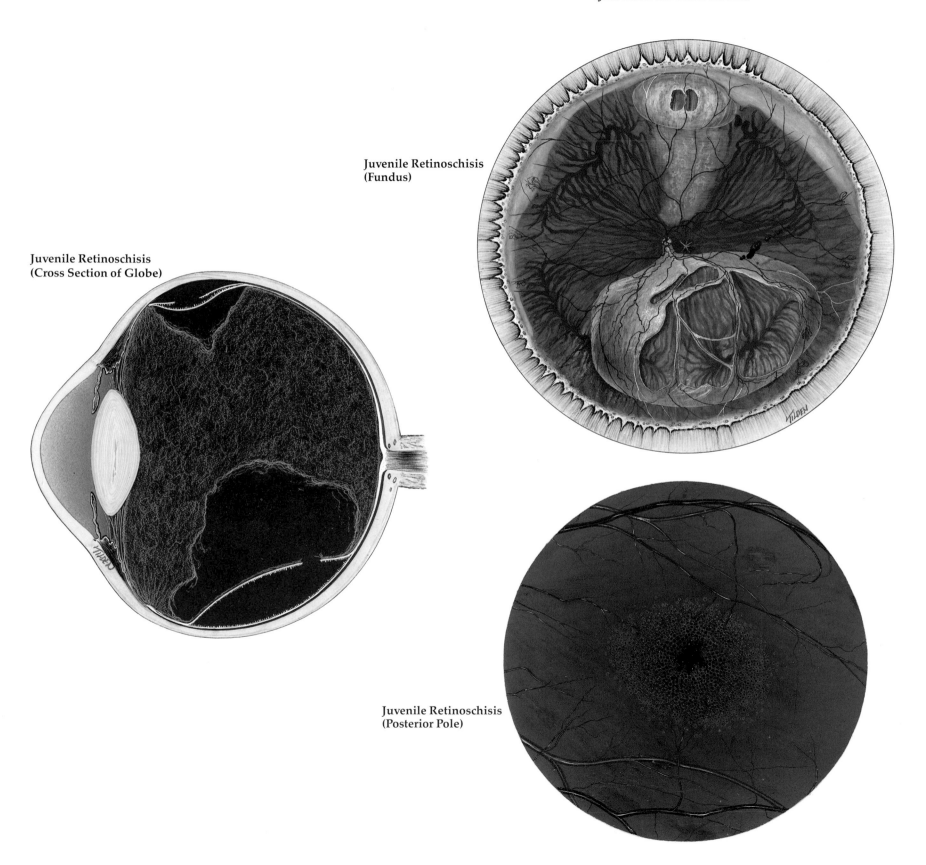

Juvenile Retinoschisis
(Fundus)

Juvenile Retinoschisis
(Cross Section of Globe)

Juvenile Retinoschisis
(Posterior Pole)

Goldmann-Favre Disease

Goldmann-Favre disease is characterized by peripheral and macular retinoschisis, retinitis pigmentosa-like retinal changes, an optically empty vitreous cavity with vitreous veils, radial lattice degeneration, night blindness, and cataracts (see Table 6.4). Goldmann-Favre's disease is inherited as an autosomal recessive trait and therefore affects males and females equally. The disease tends to be bilateral.

The peripheral (outer and inner layer holes) and macular retinoschisis as well as the pigmentary macular (beaten metal appearance) changes in Goldmann-Favre's disease closely resemble those described for congenital retinoschisis and are responsible for constricted visual fields and poor central vision (scotomas). The "bone-corpuscle" paravascular retinal pigmentation (equator and posterior pole regions) resemble the pigmentary findings in retinitis pigmentosa. A diminished or extinct electroretinogram is also present.

The vitreous shows considerable liquefaction with a large optically empty syneresis cavity similar to that found in Wagner's vitreoretinal degeneration. Pleated vitreal membranes and a thickened posterior cortical vitreous are present, resembling a preretinal membrane. The posterior cortex is usually adherent to the inner layer of retinoschisis and to the areas of chorioretinal pigmentary proliferation. Retinal detachments in Goldmann-Favre's disease have a poor prognosis, as noted in Wagner's degeneration and in Stickler's syndrome.

Table 6.4.

Goldmann-Favre Disease: Ophthalmic Findings

Optically empty vitreous

Absent posterior cortical vitreous detachment

Thickened posterior cortical vitreous

Congenital retinoschisis picture
   Inner layer retinal holes
   Outer layer retinal holes
   Retinal detachments

Retinitis pigmentosa picture
   Paravascular retinal pigmentation
   Diminished or extinquished ERG
   Chorioretinal atrophy

Complicated cataracts

Peripheral (congenital-type) retinoschisis

Macular retinoschisis
   Macular pigment changes (beaten metal)

Constricted visual fields

Central scotomas

Bilateral disease

Autosomal recessive (familial) transmission

Goldmann-Favre Disease   **Plate 29**

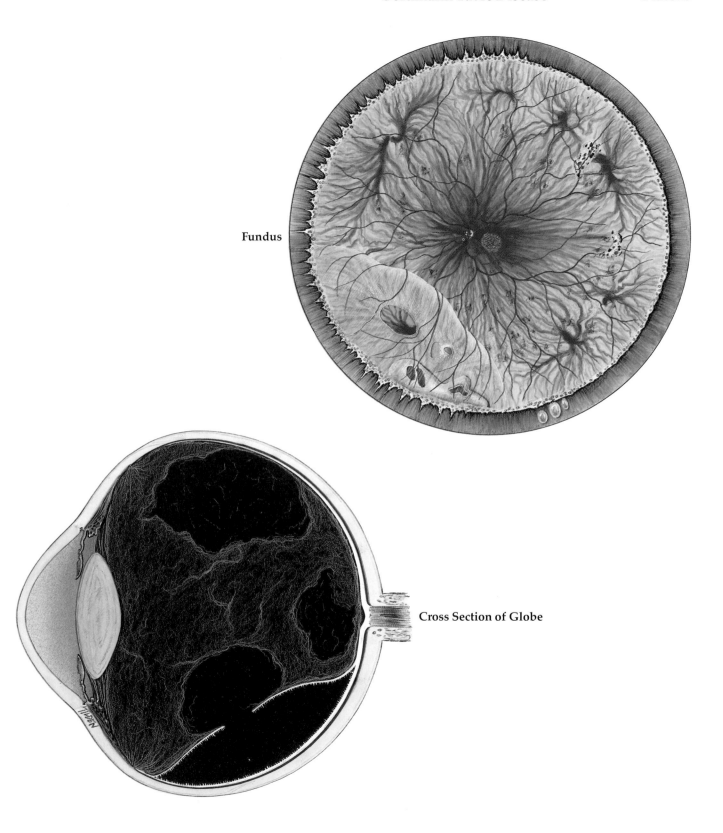

Fundus

Cross Section of Globe

Familial Exudative Vitreoretinopathy

Familial exudative vitreoretinopathy is an autosomal dominant disorder affecting young individuals who usually present with late signs, including cataract, strabismus, and nystagmus. Vitreous exudation is found throughout the vitreous gel. Vitreous contraction is the prominent feature of this disorder and there is vitreous condensation in the vitreous base and cortical regions. White-with-pressure and peripheral cystoid degeneration are often present.

Liquefaction of the vitreous gel is an infrequent finding. Posterior cortical vitreous detachments may be present, but are not found in the optic nerve head and macular regions. Contraction of the vitreous body is a constant finding. A dragged disc may also be seen. The vitreous gel has a haze, and sometimes it has a snowflake appearance. Often there is a low-grade iridocyclitis with cells in the aqueous humor and in the anterior vitreous, which are most likely due to vitreous traction on the ciliary body. Intravitreal bands can lead to retinal tears with rolled edges.

In the advanced stages of this disease, tractional retinal detachment, massive periretinal proliferation, and vitreous hemorrhage are often seen. In addition, peripheral retinal neovascularization may be responsible for recurrent vitreous hemorrhages. If a patient develops a rhegmatogenous retinal detachment, scleral buckling surgery will be required. With a vitreous hemorrhage, a pars plana vitrectomy may also be indicated, but usually the surgical results and visual prognosis in these patients are poor.

The differential diagnosis of familial exudative vitreoretinopathy includes retrolental fibroplasia, Coat's disease, Eales' disease, peripheral uveitis, angiomatosis retinae, and posterior persistent hyperplastic primary vitreous.

Familial Exudative Vitreoretinopathy   **Plate 30**

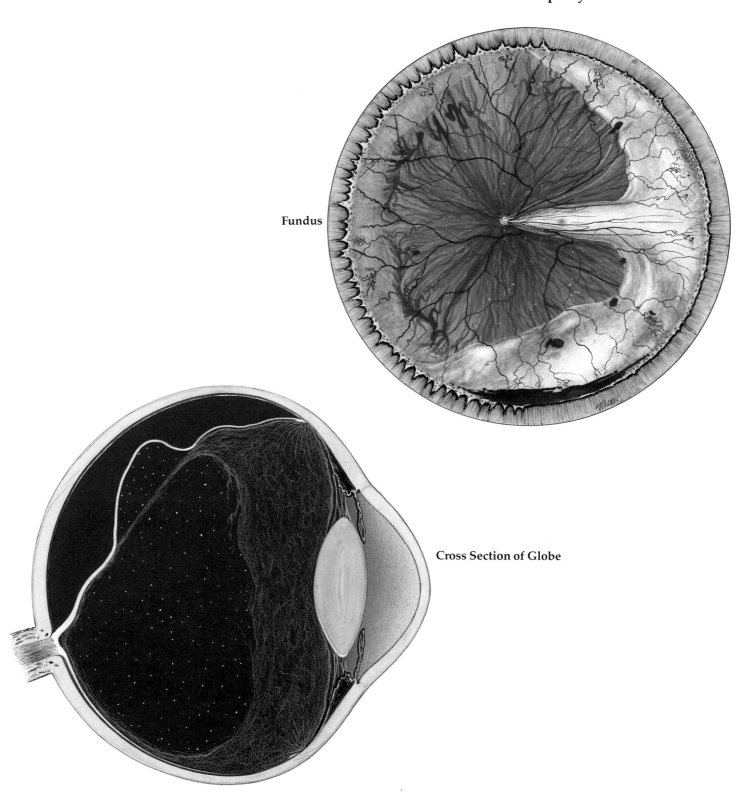

Fundus

Cross Section of Globe

Snowflake Vitreoretinal Degeneration

Snowflake hereditary vitreoretinal degeneration is a progressive disorder characterized by vitreous strands, syneresis of the vitreous, low-grade myopia, cataracts, and yellow retinal dots in areas of excessive white-with-pressure in the peripheral fundus. Retinal detachments in this disease are caused by multiple retinal breaks, usually at the equator in the temporal quadrants. The visual prognosis in these patients is often poor. Visual field depressions and reductions in the ERG scotopic b-wave amplitude as well as increased rod thresholds in dark-adaptation testing can be found in the later stages of snowflake vitreoretinal degeneration. The disease itself has been divided into the four stages listed in Table 6.5.

Table 6.5.
Snowflake Vitreoretinal Degeneration

Stage	Age (years)	Features
I	Under 15	Extensive white-with-pressure in fundus periphery
II	15–25	Minute snowflakes (yellowish dots) in areas of white-with-pressure; snowflakes are located on inner portion of neurosensory retina; decreased retinal transparency in region of snowflakes
		Snowflake distribution patterns: Anterior location — Snowflakes scattered around fundus periphery — Posterior location — Radial – paravascular — Equatorial – discrete areas parallel to the equator
		Snowflakes cratered with excavated centers (saucer-shaped) and thickened overlying vitreous
		↓ Dark adaptation (↑ rod threshold)
III	25–50	Retinal vessels are sheathed (white threads). There are pigment abnormalities (clumps of pigment) at posterior margins of snowflake craters
		Floating vitreous strands
		Cataracts
		ERG's (↓)
		Visual fields (↓)
IV	Over 60	Increased fundus pigmentation
		Retinal vessels may "disappear"
		Chorioretinal atrophy around previous pigment clumps
		Snowflakes less prominent
		Retina is atrophic; patients usually have surgical aphakia
		Night blindness

Abstracted with permission from Schepens CL: Retinal Detachment and Allied Diseases, Vol. 2, Philadelphia, W.B. Saunders Company, 1983, pp 614–615.

Snowflake Vitreoretinal Degeneration   Plate 31

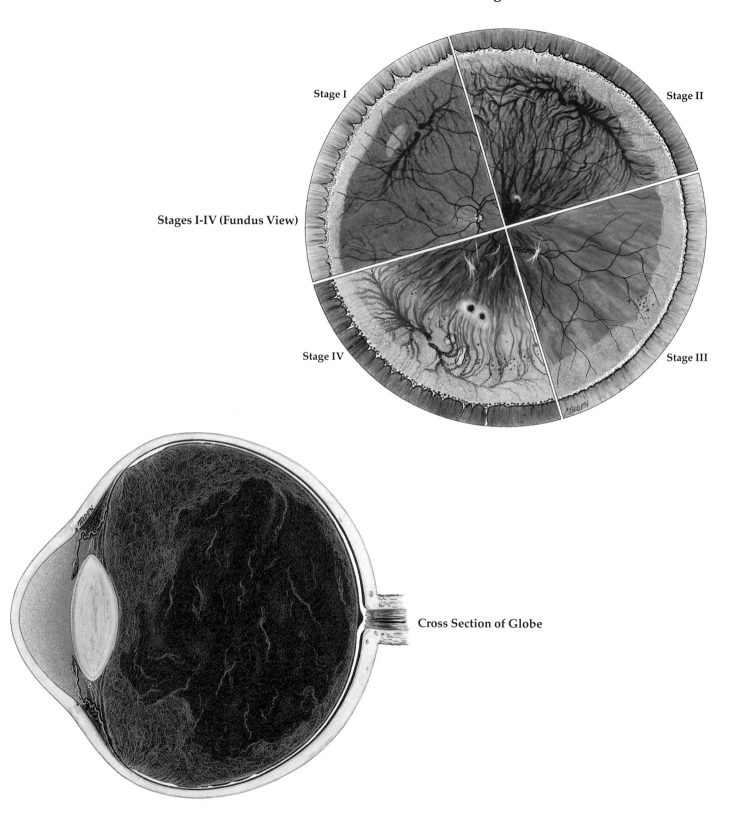

Stage I

Stage II

Stages I-IV (Fundus View)

Stage IV

Stage III

Cross Section of Globe

Systemic Conditions Associated With Vitreoretinal Degenerations

Marfan's Syndrome

Marfan's syndrome is characterized by arachnodactyly, connective tissue abnormalities such as aortic aneurysms, hypermobility of joints, and ectopia lentis. There is an autosomal dominant inheritance pattern, and males and females are affected equally. Most cases of Marfan's syndrome are caused by an inability of the tissues to incorporate hydroxyproline into specific proteins in a normal manner. In a small percentage (20%) of Marfan cases, the metabolic defect involves homocystine.

Patients with Marfan's syndrome often have high myopia and vitreous and lattice degeneration with associated retinal breaks commonly located in the equatorial region, which predispose the affected eyes to develop retinal detachments. Removal of subluxated or dislocated lenses in Marfan's patients is frequently accompanied by vitreous loss, which, in turn, further increases the chances of developing a retinal detachment. Frequently their pupils fail to dilate well, and, along with subluxation of their lenses, it is difficult to get a clear view of the retinal periphery using indirect ophthalmoscopy. Marfan's patients also have anterior chamber angle abnormalities and are predisposed to open-angle glaucoma.

Marfan's Syndrome Plate 32

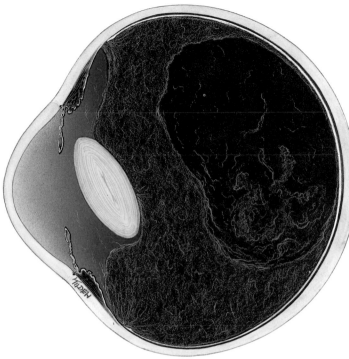

Marfan's Syndrome (Cross Section of Globe)
– Subluxated Lens

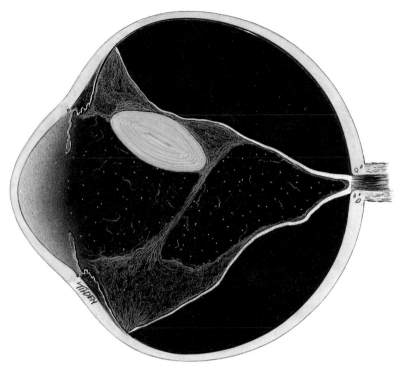

Marfan's Syndrome (Cross Section of Globe)
– Subluxated Lens with Retinal Detachment

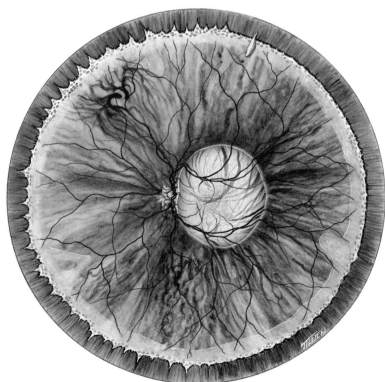

Marfan's Syndrome (Fundus)
– Myopia with Posterior Staphyloma

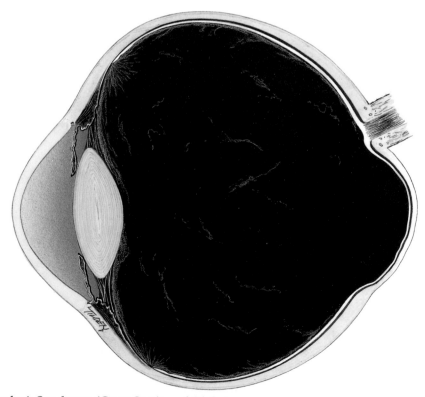

Marfan's Syndrome (Cross Section of Globe)
– Myopia with Posterior Staphyloma

Plate 33   **Homocystinuria**

Homocystinuria

In about 20% of patients with Marfan's syndrome, the metabolic defect involves inadequate homocystine incorporation into tissues, resulting in *homocystinuria* (positive nitroprusside reaction in urine). Patients with homocystinuria (autosomal recessive transmission) are often mentally deficient, whereas patients with Marfan's syndrome have normal intelligence. Also associated with homocystinuria is a tendency for cutaneous flushing and osteoporosis.

Ocular findings in homocystinuria include ectopia lentis, high myopia, lattice degeneration, and an increased tendency to develop peripheral retinal tears and retinal detachments. Removal of a subluxated lens is often accompanied by vitreous loss, which may lead to retinal detachment.

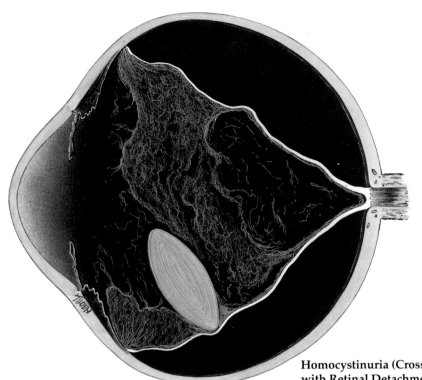

Homocystinuria (Cross Section of Globe) – Dislocated Lens with Retinal Detachment

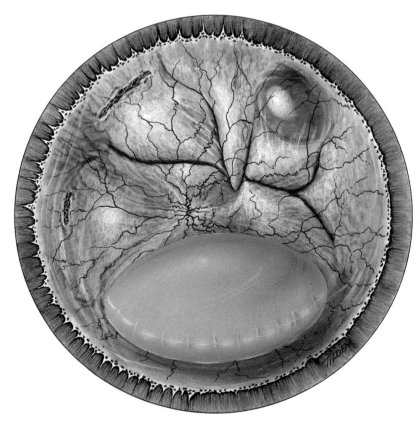

Homocystinuria (Fundus) – Dislocated Lens with Retinal Detachment

Ehlers-Danlos Syndrome

Ehlers-Danlos syndrome is an autosomal dominant inherited biochemical defect involving abnormal formation of collagen fibers. It is manifested clinically in all tissues in which collagen fibers are a main structural component. Hyperelastic and fragile skin, hyperextensibility of the joints especially in the fingers, poor wound healing, and scarring are just some of the manifestations of this connective tissue disorder.

Associated ocular findings in Ehlers-Danlos syndrome include ptosis, hypotony of the extrinsic ocular muscles – often leading to strabismus, Méténier's sign (unusual ease in everting the upper eyelid), epicanthus, myopia, blue sclera, keratoconus, and ectopia lentis.

Vitreoretinal findings in Ehlers-Danlos syndrome include angioid streaks, macular degeneration, equatorial pigmentary degeneration, and retinal breaks (temporal quadrants) with strong vitreoretinal traction forces present. Rolled edges are very often present at the retinal tear sites, along with areas of white-without-pressure. Premature vitreous degeneration (including collapse of the vitreous gel), vitreous hemorrhage, and retinal detachments are associated with Ehlers-Danlos syndrome.

Ehlers-Danlos Syndrome **Plate 34**

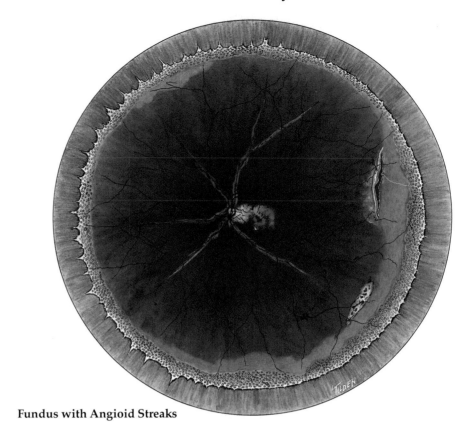

Fundus with Angioid Streaks

Cross Section of Globe with Retinal Detachment

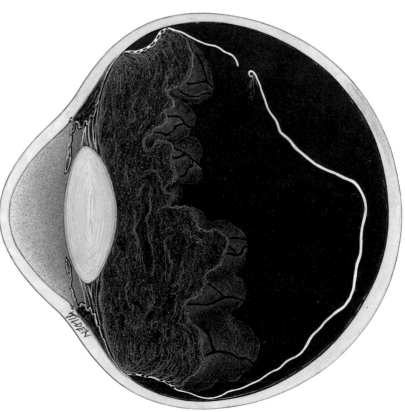

Degenerative Conditions of the Vitreous Body

7

Asteroid Hyalosis
Synchysis Scintillans (Cholesterolosis Oculi)
Amyloidosis of the Vitreous

Plate 35   **Asteroid Hyalosis**

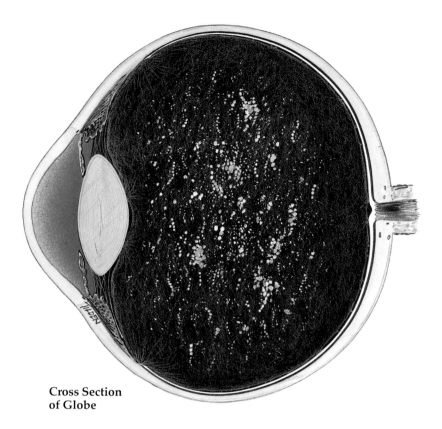

**Cross Section
of Globe**

Asteroid Hyalosis

Asteroid hyalosis is characterized by the presence of white spherical particles embedded in the vitreous body. About 27% of patients with asteroid hyalosis are diabetic, yet only 5.4% of diabetic patients have asteroid hyalosis. Therefore, the findings of asteroid hyalosis should alert the examiner to the possibility of diabetes in the patient. Asteroid hyalosis is unilateral in 75% of cases. There is no special sexual or racial predilection. Asteroid hyalosis is usually asymptomatic even in cases where the particles are so numerous that it is difficult to see the retina with indirect ophthalmoscopy. Yet many of the patients do not report decreased visual acuity! The reasons for this discrepancy are not clear.

Biomicroscopically, the yellow-white bodies are characteristically trapped in the anterior and central vitreous gel. They are rarely located in liquefied vitreous, Cloquet's canal, or the retrovitreous space. The asteroid particles are often located along fibrous strands of the vitreous accounting for their "string-of-pearls" appearance. One important feature of the particles in asteroid hyalosis is that, after eye movement, they return to their original position in the vitreous cavity. In contrast, the particles in synchysis scintillans do not return to their original position after eye movements or a change in body position or gravity.

Histopathology studies indicate that asteroid hyalosis bodies are calcium soaps of degenerating vitreous fibers and are associated with a type of foreign body giant cell reaction. The central cores of these particles are birefringent when viewed with polarized light, whereas the capsule or outer portion is not birefringent and appears to be made up of condensed vitreous fibrils. The asteroid particles stain positively with lipid stains (oil red O, Sudan black) and with acid mucopolysaccharide stains (Alcian blue, colloidal iron).

Asteroid hyalosis seldom requires treatment, since it usually is asymptomatic. However, in rare cases it may be responsible for profound visual loss, especially if there is an extremely dense concentration of the particles in the central vitreous cavity. Pars plana vitrectomy can be used to remove the central asteroid bodies and restore vision in these severe cases.

Synchysis Scintillans (Cholesterolosis Oculi)

Synchysis scintillans is a degenerative condition where cholesterol crystals are deposited in the vitreous, in the anterior chamber, and in the subretinal space. This is a relatively rare condition, but it is usually secondary to ocular trauma, chronic recurrent intraocular hemorrhage, or inflammation.

Patients usually do not complain of visual symptoms from the vitreous opacities because the vision is extremely poor in that eye, either from a retinal detachment or a cataract. If iridocyclitis or glaucoma occurs as a result of cholesterolosis of the anterior chamber (resembles a hypopyon), then the patient may experience ocular pain.

Ophthalmoscopy reveals numerous multicolored glittering crystalline particles whose size and shape are quite variable. With ocular movement they are dispersed and resemble multicolored confetti and then settle by gravity when eye movement stops. Biomicroscopy shows extensive liquefaction of the vitreous in synchysis scintillans. The particles are flat with angular edges and are multicolored.

Microscopic examination indicates that most of the crystals are cholesterol, although tyrosine, leucine, and margarine crystals have also been found. The origin of the crystalline particles in synchysis scintillans remains obscure. One hypothesis suggests that a cholesterol-fatty acid-ester combination in the blood is the source. Once inside the eye, the molecule breaks down, releasing free cholesterol and fatty acids. Since free cholesterol is highly insoluble, it crystallizes out of solution. Another theory suggests that the crystalline particles may originate from a lens that is ruptured secondary to trauma. As for treatment, patients with synchysis scintillans usually do not require treatment unless the particles clog the aqueous drainage system, resulting in glaucoma. In such cases, the particles are irrigated from the anterior chamber.

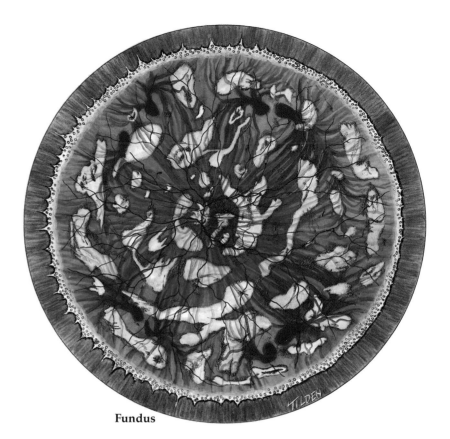

Fundus

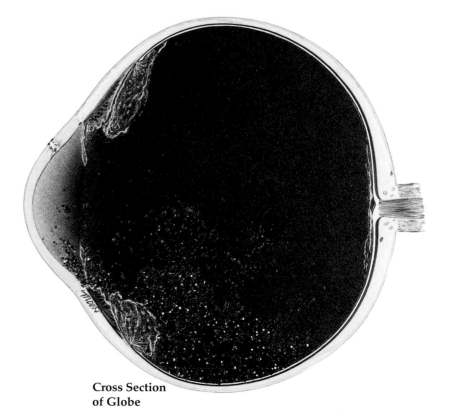

**Cross Section
of Globe**

Amyloidosis of the Vitreous

Primary amyloidosis involves the deposition of amyloid material along collagen fibers and usually involves the heart, pancreas, thyroid, eye, peripheral nerves, and muscles and is not associated with debilitating diseases. *Secondary amyloidosis* involves the deposition of amyloid material along reticulin fibers and usually involves the liver, spleen, adrenal glands, and kidney and is associated with chronic debilitating diseases such as neoplasms, metabolic disorders, infectious and noninfectious chronic inflammations, and dysproteinemias.

Primary heredofamilial amyloidosis involves ocular tissues and is transmitted as a simple Mendelian dominant trait. Elevations of the β_1- and α_2-lipoprotein fractions seem to suggest that an anomaly of lipoprotein metabolism may be present in primary amyloidosis.

Systemic manifestations of primary amyloidosis include weight loss, generalized weakness, and progressive peripheral neuropathy, as well as cardiovascular, gastrointestinal, and endocrine disorders. Symptoms appear usually by the second decade.

Ocular involvement is found in 8% of patients with primary amyloidosis and can be manifested by photophobia, sudden loss of vision, diplopia, blepharospasm, external ophthalmoplegia, and sluggish pupils, as well as "cotton-wool" retinal exudates and vitreous opacities (see Table 7.1).

Early ophthalmoscopic changes seen in the fundus consist of a whitish lesion in the wall of a retinal arteriole, which develops cottonlike fringes in the vitreous cortex. Then the paravascular "cotton-wool" spot spreads out and grows into the vitreous cavity. As the opacities become denser, they obscure the underlying retinal architecture. Amyloid deposits can cover the disc and macular region and be responsible for a marked decrease in central vision. The affected vitreous gel has a "glass-wool" appearance to it. When a posterior vitreous detachment takes place, the amyloid deposits may detach from the retinal surface and shift position. Sometimes these amyloid deposits become displaced along the visual axis, thereby reducing vision.

The differential diagnosis of these amyloid vitreous opacities should include inflammatory vitreous exudates from chorioretinitic foci or pars planitis. Usually there are chorioretinal foci that identify the source of the vitreous exudate. Pars planitis has exudates in the pars plana as well as in the vitreous, whereas amyloidosis does not have a pars plana "exudate." Other differential diagnostic possibilities include an organized vitreous hemorrhage, which, if old, has a membranous, dirty white-yellow appearance. Usually, there are some unresolved red blood clots, and with time these tend to melt away or clear partially, whereas amyloidosis is relentlessly progressive. Retained intraocular metallic foreign bodies and parasitic foreign bodies have a membranous quality to them, often with a hemorrhagic element, which is not characteristic of amyloidosis.

Table 7.1.

Primary Heredofamilial Amyloidosis

Ocular symptoms
- Diplopia
- Photophobia
- Progressive loss of vision
- Sudden loss of vision

Ocular signs
- Blepharospasm
- Bilateral exophthalmos
- External ophthalmoplegia
- Anisocoria
- Sluggish pupillary reflexes
- Retinal hemorrhages
- Paravascular retinal exudates (amyloid)
  - "Cotton-wool" exudates
- Blood vessel wall deposits (amyloid)
  - Central retinal artery
  - Short posterior ciliary vessels
- Vitreous changes
  - Both eyes affected
  - Vitreous opacities ("glass-wool")

Amyloidosis of the Vitreous   **Plate 37**

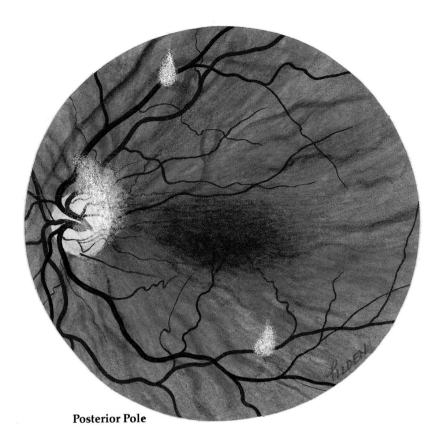

Posterior Pole

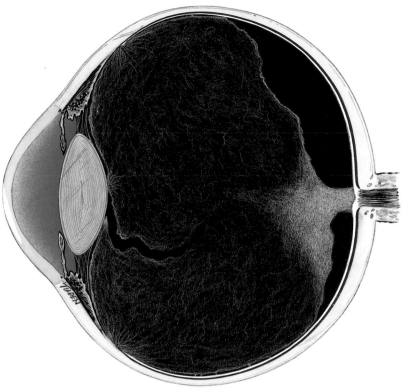

Cross Section of Globe through Optic Disc

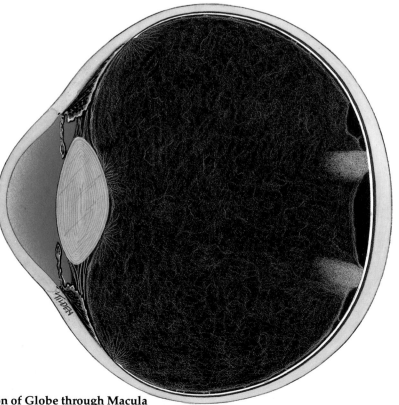

Cross Section of Globe through Macula

Proliferative Retinopathies 8

Diabetic Retinopathy

Diabetes mellitus is a genetically determined metabolic disorder characterized clinically by elevated fasting blood sugars, arteriosclerotic and microangiopathic vasculopathies and neuropathies. The exact pathogenic sequence of diabetic retinopathy has yet to be worked out, but it appears that the elevated blood sugars and decreased plasma insulin levels influence the pituitary gland to manufacture and release increased amounts of human growth hormone into the plasma. The increased growth hormone potentiates hepatic protein synthesis of α_2-globulins and fibrinogen. These macromolecules act as electrostatic bridges between neighboring red blood cells and platelets resulting in abnormal red blood cells as well as platelet aggregates. These abnormal aggregates clog up capillary channels leading to downstream hypoxia and, in some cases, ischemia. Microaneurysms (aborted attempts at neovascularization) and actual retinal and/or optic disc neovascularization may develop in an effort to correct the hypoxia problems in the retinal tissues.

The overall incidence of diabetes mellitus involves about 5% of the general population. Of all known diabetics, 8% are less than 25 years of age when the diagnosis is made; 22% are diagnosed between the ages of 25 and 44 years, and 50% are diagnosed between the ages of 45 and 64 years of age; 20% of diabetics are diagnosed after 65 years of age. Approximately 50% of all diabetics will have some form of retinopathy at the time that their diabetes is diagnosed, and it is related to age of onset and duration of the diabetes mellitus. The overall incidence of proliferative diabetic retinopathy is 4.4% of all diabetics. Surprisingly, there is a higher incidence of proliferative diabetic retinopathy among non-insulin-dependent diabetics than among insulin-dependent diabetics.

Diabetic retinopathy can be divided into three separate stages: (1) background (nonproliferative) retinopathy, (2) preproliferative retinopathy, and (3) proliferative retinopathy.

Background Diabetic Retinopathy

Background diabetic retinopathy is characterized by an initial dilation in the retinal veins, retinal microaneurysms, dot-blot or deep round retinal hemorrhages, and/or deep hard waxy retinal exudates. Microaneurysms and retinal vessels may leak, producing localized or diffuse retinal edema, including macular edema with concomitant visual loss. Background diabetic retinopathy predominantly affects the posterior pole.

Preproliferative Diabetic Retinopathy

The preproliferative stage of diabetic retinopathy usually consists of cotton-wool spots in addition to the background diabetic retinopathy changes already described. The cotton-wool spot represents hypoxia and/or ischemia in the inner surface of the retina at the nerve fiber layer. Eventually, there is resolution or clearing of the cotton-wool spot, but often at the edge of the cotton-wool spot, neovascularization of the retina may develop. For these reasons, the cotton-wool spot stage (unrelated to systemic hypertension) in a diabetic is referred to as the preproliferative stage. In addition, retinal venous beading and intraretinal microvascular abnormalities (IRMA), which refer to dilated retinal capillary shunt vessels around areas of capillary bed nonperfusion (fluorescein angiographic finding) may also be present.

Proliferative Diabetic Retinopathy

In the proliferative stage, retinal and/or disc neovascularization has taken place in addition to the preproliferative retinopathy findings already present. The new blood vessels grow and may progress to a point where there is connective tissue or glial proliferation that accompanies the neovascularization process. The new vessels may grow into and become adherent to the vitreous body. In some cases, there is spontaneous regression of the neovascularization network with contracture of the connective tissue components, and this may lead to secondary vitreous hemorrhage, vitreous membranes, and a traction or a rhegmatogenous retinal detachment. These reactions may still take place without any regression of the neovascularization and connective tissue networks. Repeated vitreous hemorrhages can lead to more vitreoretinal membranes with further traction and vitreous hemorrhage in a vicious cycle (retinitis proliferans) leading to total retinal detachment, blindness and phthisis bulbi.

Leaking retinal microaneurysms in the macular region have been treated with either focal or grid pattern argon laser photocoagulation to control macular edema and stabilize vision. Pan retinal argon laser photocoagulation has been successful in controlling proliferative diabetic retinopathy and reducing the chances of intraocular hemorrhage in early cases. Pars plana vitrectomy and scleral buckling surgery have helped restore vision in advanced cases of proliferative diabetic retinopathy with nonresolving vitreous hemorrhages and with tractional retinal detachments.

Diabetic Retinopathy   **Plate 38**

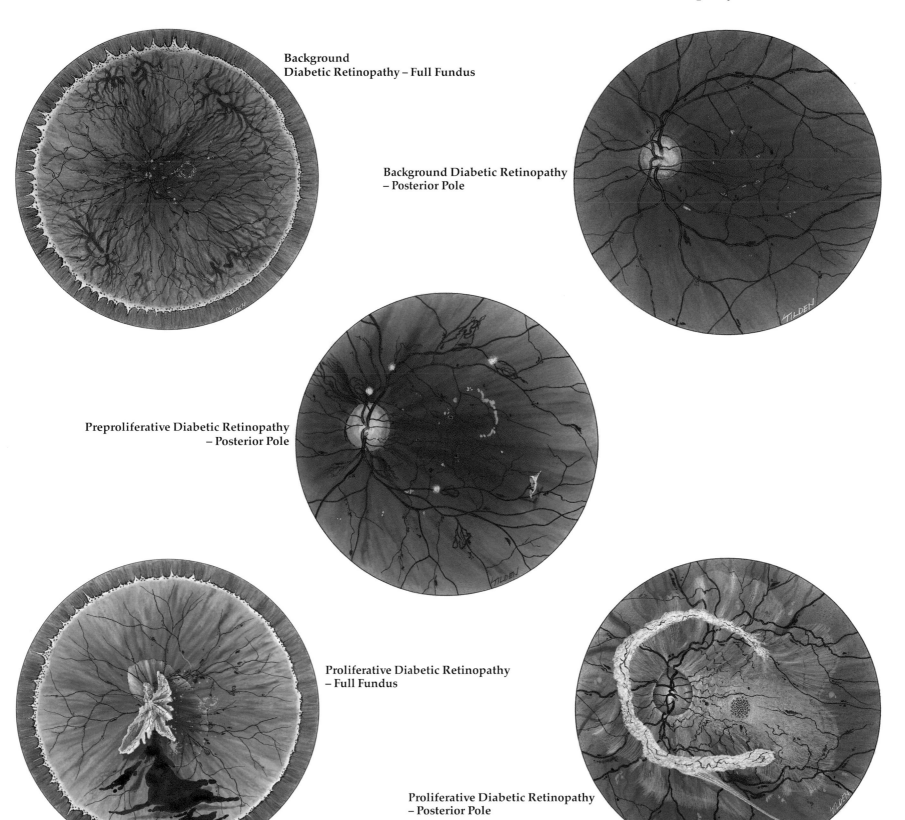

Background
Diabetic Retinopathy – Full Fundus

Background Diabetic Retinopathy
– Posterior Pole

Preproliferative Diabetic Retinopathy
– Posterior Pole

Proliferative Diabetic Retinopathy
– Full Fundus

Proliferative Diabetic Retinopathy
– Posterior Pole

Retinal Vein Occlusion

Retinal vein occlusions are usually due to arteriosclerosis and systemic hypertension. Among branch retinal vein occlusions, the superotemporal branch (63%) is more commonly affected than the inferotemporal branch retinal vein (38%). This increased incidence of the superotemporal branch retinal vein occluding correlates with its larger number of arteriovenous crossings (3) compared to the arteriovenous crossings (2) in the other quadrants.

Characteristically, an acute branch retinal vein occlusion has superficial splinter retinal hemorrhages, deep round retinal hemorrhages, as well as widened and more tortuous retinal veins in the sector of the obstruction. Retinal edema, including macular edema (58%) with concomitant reduction in visual acuity, is often present. On occasion, cotton-wool spots may also be noted as well as retinal microaneurysms. Other adverse macular sequelae include macular hole formation, surface wrinkling retinopathy, granularity and/or hyperpigmentation of the retinal pigment epithelium, macular exudates, detachments, and hemorrhage. In the later stages, intraretinal neovascularization (73%), preretinal neovascularization (23%), and secondary vitreous hemorrhage (20%) may develop, which, in turn, could lead to vitreoretinal membranes and a possible traction and/or rhegmatogenous retinal detachment. Eyes with retinal vein occlusions that have wide areas of capillary bed nonperfusion are more likely to develop retinal and/or optic disc neovascularization. Eyes with central retinal vein occlusions are more likely to develop neovascularization than those with branch retinal vein occlusions. Also, patients who develop optic disc and/or retinal neovascularization may go on to acquire rubeosis iridis with hemorrhagic glaucoma. Aphakic eyes are more prone to this complication than phakic eyes. Compensatory vascular reactions to the vein occlusion involve the development of various collaterals, for example, vein to vein.

Retinal Vein Occlusion **Plate 39**

Central Retinal Vein Occlusion – Fundus

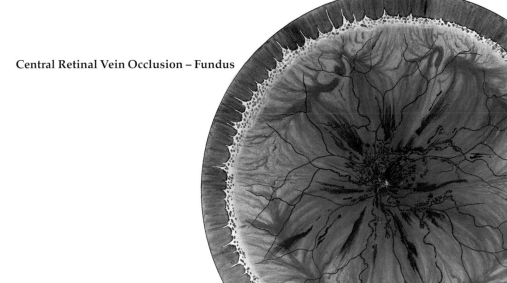

Central Retinal Vein Occlusion – Posterior Pole

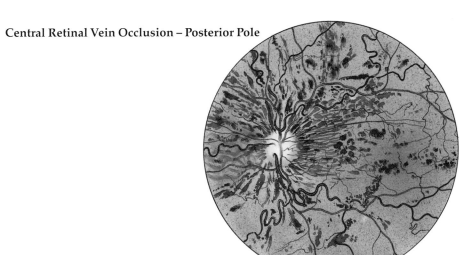

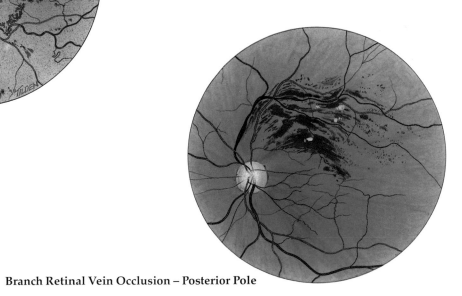

Branch Retinal Vein Occlusion – Posterior Pole

Sickle Cell Retinopathy

Hemoglobin S has the tendency to become insoluble and turn to a gel when deoxygenated, leading to highly abnormal viscous aggregates of sickled (crescent-shaped) red blood cells, which, in turn, may cause vascular obstruction. The abnormal hemoglobins in this family include SS, SC, and AS.

Ophthalmoscopically, sickle cell retinopathy usually presents with dilated tortuous retinal veins, and discoid-shaped retinal scars, which have been termed the "black sunburst" sign. Patients with Hb-SC disease have characteristic equatorial arteriovenous vascular shunts projecting into the vitreous termed "sea fans." Vitreous hemorrhages often accompany patients with sea fans, and this can go on to the formation of vitreoretinal membranes with traction and/or rhegmatogenous retinal detachments. Sickle cell patients with hemoglobin SC retinopathy have been divided by Goldberg (1971) into five separate clinical stages, which, in some cases, are progressive (Table 8.1).

Table 8.1.

Proliferative Sickle Cell (Hb-SC) Retinopathy

Stage	Features
I	Peripheral arteriolar occlusions
II	Peripheral arteriolar-venular anastamoses (sea fans)
III	Neovascular and fibrous proliferations
IV	Vitreous hemorrhage
V	Retinal detachment

Reprinted with permission from Goldberg MF: Classification and pathogenesis of proliferative sickle retinopathy. Ophthalmology 71: 649–665. Philadelphia, Lippincott/Harper & Row, 1971

Proliferative Sickle Cell Retinopathy   **Plate 40**

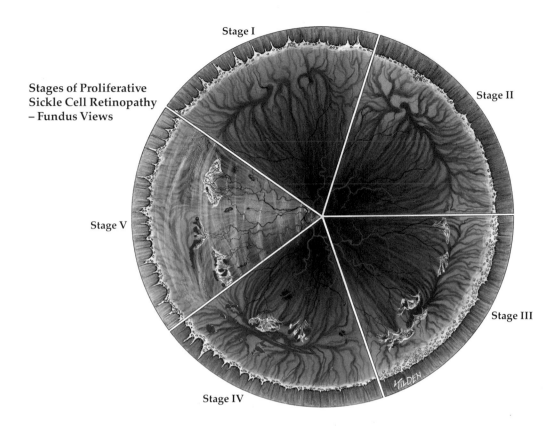

Stages of Proliferative Sickle Cell Retinopathy – Fundus Views

Stage I

Stage II

Stage III

Stage IV

Stage V

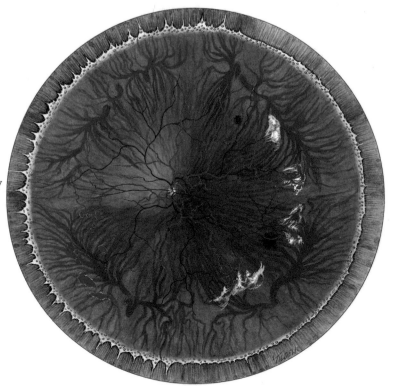

Proliferative Sickle Cell Retinopathy – Stage IV (Fundus)

Retrolental Fibroplasia

Retrolental fibroplasia (RLF) is usually seen when premature infants are treated with "too much oxygen" for respiratory distress. Rarely does RLF occur in full-term infants that are given oxygen therapy. The reasons for this are that premature infants do not have a completely developed or mature retinal vasculature in the retinal periphery, especially in the temporal quadrants compared to the nasal quadrants. The immature retinal vasculature is susceptible to the effects of high concentrations of oxygen, which provoke an initial vasoconstriction followed by retinal neovascularization and the development of RLF. In full-term infants, the retinal vasculature is "mature" and does not undergo the proliferative reactions in the presence of elevated concentrations of oxygen.

The development of retinal vessels begins at the optic disc at about the fourth month of gestation and reaches the ora serrata by the eighth month of gestation. The distance from the optic nerve head to the ora serrata in the temporal quadrants is greater than the distance from the optic disc to the ora serrata in the nasal quadrants. There is greater immaturity of the temporal retinal periphery than the nasal retinal periphery during the gestational period, which may be the reason that in premature infants treated with excessive oxygen there is a predilection for RLF to be found in temporal quadrants as opposed to nasal quadrants.

The precise mechanism by which oxygen leads to vaso-obliteration of the immature retinal capillaries is not known. However, it is believed that high oxygen concentrations are toxic to actively growing capillary endothelial cells, which leads, in some way, to obliteration of the developing capillary bed. Once obliteration occurs, proliferative neovascular tissues develop, leading to acute retrolental fibroplasia. In some cases there is spontaneous regression, in others, a cicatricial phase follows with varying amounts of tissue damage, including vitreoretinal membranes, exudative, traction, and/or rhegmatogenous retinal detachments. Retrolental fibroplasia eyes also have a characteristic high myopia, congenital nystagmus, amblyopia, and strabismus. The various stages of retrolental fibroplasia are listed in Table 8.2.

Table 8.2.

Stages of Retrolental Fibroplasia

Stage	Ocular Findings
Acute Phase	Vaso-obliterative (while on O_2)
	Vasoproliferative (after O_2 is discontinued)
	Large arteriovenous shunt + proliferative capillaries
	Spontaneous regression (80%)
Chronic Phase (Cicatricial 20%)[1]	
Grade I	Myopia
	Retinal pigmentation
	Vitreous membranes
	Equatorial retinal folds
Grade II	Grade I plus:
	Dragging of the retina
	Ectopic macula
	Neovascularization
	Elevated retinal vessels
	Lattice degeneration
	Retinal breaks
Grade III	Falciform retinal folds
	Amblyopia
	Ocular nystagmus
Grade IV	Rhegmatogenous retinal detachment
	Tractional exudative retinal detachment
Grade V	Organized retinal detachment

[1] Reprinted with permission from Tasman W: Late complications of retrolental fibroplasia. Ophthalmology 86 (10): 1724–40. Philadelphia, Lippincott/Harper & Row, 1979

Retrolental Fibroplasia **Plate 41**

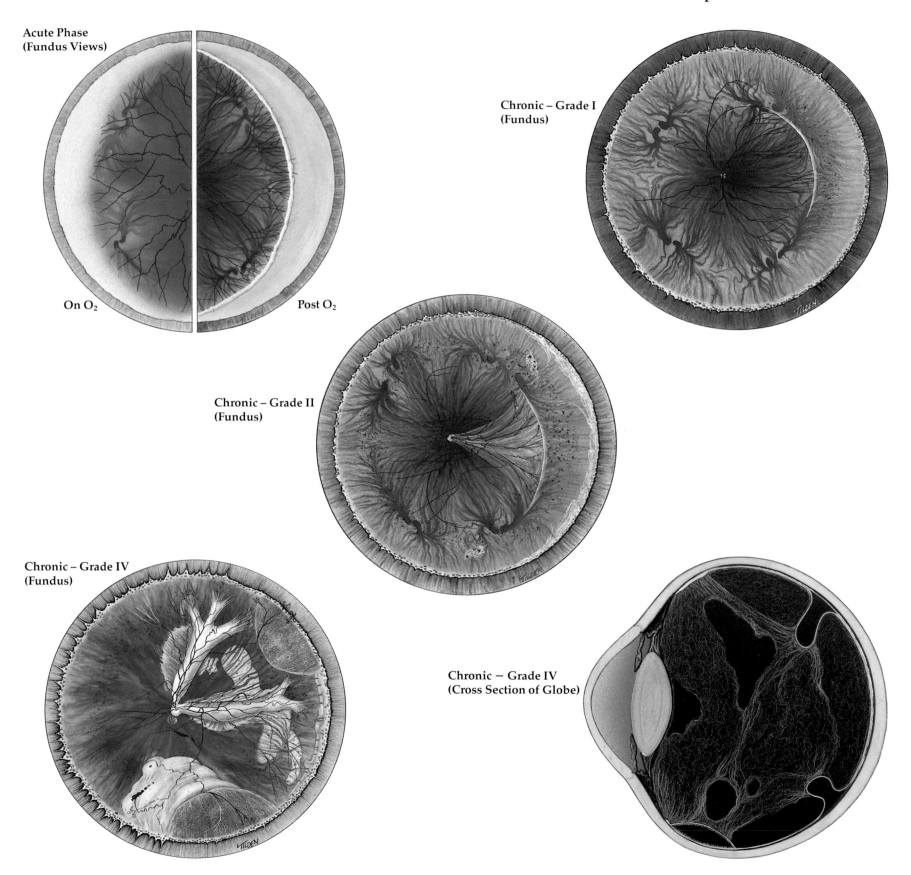

Acute Phase
(Fundus Views)

On O₂

Post O₂

Chronic – Grade I
(Fundus)

Chronic – Grade II
(Fundus)

Chronic – Grade IV
(Fundus)

Chronic – Grade IV
(Cross Section of Globe)

Inflammatory Disorders 9

Plate 42   **Sarcoidosis**

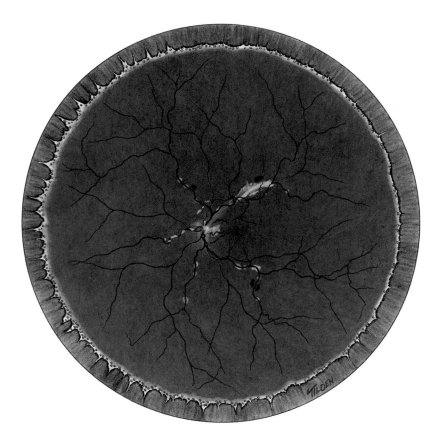

Sarcoidosis

Sarcoidosis is an inflammatory disorder of unknown origin more common in blacks than in whites and is characterized by fever, arthritis, lymphadenopathy, central nervous system as well as ocular lesions. The basic lesion consists of a focal noncaseating granuloma containing nodular collections of epithelioid cells.

Ocular manifestations of sarcoidosis include conjunctival nodules, a granulomatous uveitis (anterior and/or posterior), and retinal as well as optic nerve involvement. A retinal periphlebitis along with retinal hemorrhages, vitreous veils, and intraretinal and subretinal pigment epithelium granulomas may be present. There is a perivascular collection of lymphocytes along the retinal veins, which have periphlebitis. Intense retinal periphlebitis, in sarcoidosis, may produce the typical appearance of "candle-wax drippings" which have a predilection for the retinal veins within the posterior pole. Small superficial retinal hemorrhages may also be noted. In some cases, there is diffuse choroidal involvement leading to focal pigmentary atrophy and scarring.

Sarcoidosis that involves the central nervous system may also affect the optic nerve producing a picture of papillitis and papilledema.

Harada's Syndrome
(Vogt-Koyanagi-Harada Syndrome)

Harada's syndrome is an inflammatory disorder of unknown etiology that affects young adult blacks, orientals, and darkly pigmented Caucasians. There is no particular sexual predilection, with males and females equally affected. Patients may present with headaches, nausea, tinnitus, and general malaise. Meningeal irritation can be responsible for cerebrospinal pleocytosis and a stiff neck. In the later stages of the disease, poliosis and alopecia are seen.

Ocular findings consist of a bilateral granulomatous uveitis, ocular pain, redness, and photophobia, with a number of inflammatory cells found in the aqueous and vitreous. There are often multiple dome-shaped exudative detachments of the neurosensory retina. There is retinal edema, and, on occasion, some retinal hemorrhages may be present. The shifting subretinal fluid may be clear or turbid. In some cases, the multiple retinal detachment sites coalesce into a large retinal detachment due to the effects of gravity. Typically, no retinal tears are present. The source of the subretinal fluid is not well established, but histopathologic analysis of eyes with Harada's syndrome reveals a diffuse granulomatous uveitis involving the choriocapillaris similar to that of sympathetic uveitis.

Some patients with Harada's syndrome respond to systemic steroids. In others, a spontaneous resolution of the inflammatory process takes place with reattachment of the retina, leaving focal areas of retinal pigmentary atrophy.

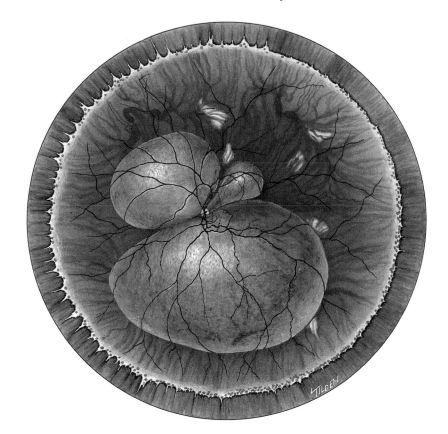

Plate 44   **Pars Planitis**

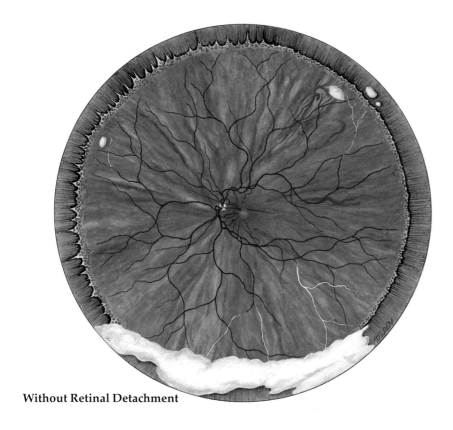

Without Retinal Detachment

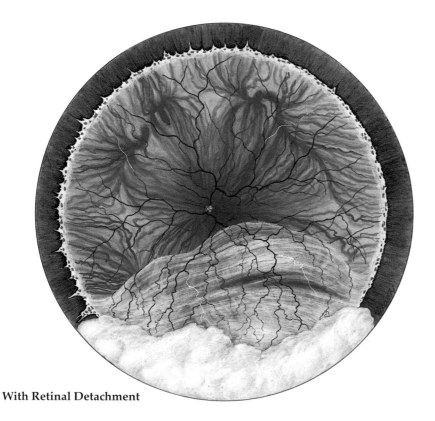

With Retinal Detachment

Pars Planitis (Idiopathic Peripheral Uveoretinitis)

Pars planitis is a chronic inflammatory process of unknown etiology affecting the peripheral fundus (retina and choroid) and the ciliary body. It tends to occur at any age, but is most severe in children and young adults. There is no particular sexual predilection with males and females equally affected by the disease. The disease is bilateral in 95% of cases and is thought by some investigators to involve a special hypersensitivity reaction to the small retinal vessels in the fundus periphery.

Ocular findings in idiopathic peripheral uveoretinitis include decreased visual acuity, normotensive or hypotensive globes, and aqueous flare with several nongranulomatous keratic precipitates, along with inflammatory cells in the anterior vitreous. White exudates (snow banks) are noted mostly inferiorly in the region of the pars plana and the vitreous base. The peripheral retinal veins appear dilated, and on occasion have perivascular infiltrates. There is often cystoid macular edema in the more severe cases.

Pars planitis tends to be a chronic condition with remissions and exacerbations. However, there is a smoldering inflammation, which leads to adverse sequelae, for example, peripheral anterior synechiae, posterior subcapsular cataracts, organization of the vitreous with vitreoretinal membranes, and traction on peripheral retinal tissues, leading to traction and/or rhegmatogenous retinal detachments and, in some cases, retinoschisis. In addition, glaucoma, band keratopathy, and dense cataracts may lead to further visual loss and blindness.

Choroidal Detachments (Ciliochoroidal Effusion)

Choroidal Detachment **Plate 45**

Choroidal detachments represent an accumulation of fluid within the suprachoroidal space (outermost layer of the choroid) and the supraciliaris space (outermost layer of the ciliary body). Although there is a detachment of the uveal tract from the inner layer of the sclera, choroidal detachments actually represent fluid accumulation within the uveal tract.

Characteristically, choroidal detachments have a brown-orange coloration, are solid-appearing elevations under intact retinal pigment epithelium and choroidal tissue layers. Choroidal detachments do not undulate with ocular movements like rhegmatogenous retinal detachments, and they do not shift under gravitational influences as do exudative retinal detachments of the neurosensory retina.

Most choroidal detachments contain serous fluid, but some are due to a choroidal hemorrhage. On occasion, a solid choroidal detachment containing tumor tissue, for example, melanoma, may be present, but ultrasonography usually can clear up the nature (solid, serous, or hemorrhagic) of the choroidal detachment.

Choroidal detachments are often due to ocular surgery or trauma to the globe where inflammation and/or hypotony are created initially, and then choroidal detachments develop secondarily. In the other cases, there is an initial rhegmatogenous retinal detachment that creates ocular hypotony, which in turn leads to the development of choroidal detachments. Once the ciliary body detaches, aqueous humor production is reduced, leading to more hypotony, which in turn leads to increased choroidal detachments. Retinal detachments that have choroidal detachments present usually have a greater chance of developing proliferative vitreoretinopathy (massive periretinal proliferation), and, in general, have a poorer visual prognosis than rhegmatogenous retinal detachments that do not have associated choroidal detachments.

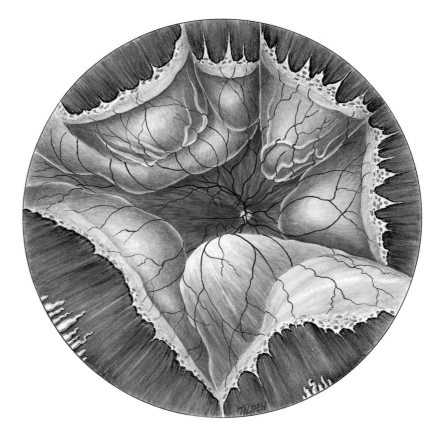

Plate 46   **Choroidal Effusion Syndrome**

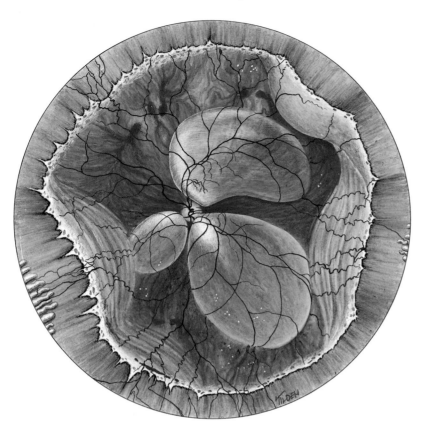

Choroidal Effusion Syndrome

The choroidal effusion syndrome is characterized by non-rhegmatogenous retinal detachment with shifting subretinal fluid, choroidal detachments, and an associated increased protein content in the cerebrospinal fluid. The patients are usually in their fifth or sixth decades of life and males and females are equally affected. The patients respond to systemic steroids, but do very poorly with scleral buckling surgery.

The differential diagnosis of the choroidal effusion syndrome detachments includes the following conditions: rhegmatogenous retinal detachments, choroidal tumors, metastatic tumors to the choroid, choroidal hemangiomas, vitreous hemorrhage, and subretinal pigment epithelial hemorrhage, and reactive lymphoid hyperplasia of the uveal tract.

Pigmentary Tumors of the Peripheral Retina

10

Choroidal Nevi
Congenital Hypertrophy of the Retinal Pigment Epithelium
Congenital Grouped Pigmentation ("Bear Tracks")
Metastatic Tumors to the Choroid
Choroidal Melanomas

Choroidal Nevi

Choroidal nevi are usually flat, well-circumscribed lesions that vary in color from brown to grey to black and vary between 0.5 disc diameters to 8 disc diameters in size. Most choroidal nevi are considered flat, but on occasion may be up to 2 mm in thickness. The edges of choroidal nevi can be sharply demarcated or feathery.

Although choroidal nevi are considered to be benign lesions, they may be responsible for a variety of changes in overlying tissues, including degeneration of the retinal pigment epithelium, and photoreceptor cells (including visual field defects), drusen formation, cystoid retinal degeneration, subretinal neovascularization with serous and hemorrhagic detachments of the neurosensory retina. On occasion, subretinal exudates are noted in a circinate pattern. Orange pigment, that is, lipofuscin seen in malignant melanomas can also be noted in some choroidal nevi.

Choroidal nevi tend to grow most rapidly during adolescence and obtain their deepest pigmentation in adulthood. About 30% of adults have choroidal nevi with a 1 in 5000 chance that the nevus will transform into a malignant melanoma. There is no particular sexual predilection for choroidal nevi, but their incidence is higher in Caucasians than in blacks.

Congenital Hypertrophy of the Retinal Pigment Epithelium

Congenital hypertrophy of the retinal pigment epithelium (CHRPE) is a discoid flat-shaped lesion at the level of the retinal pigment epithelium. It may occur as a single lesion or it may occur in a multifocal form termed *congenital grouped pigmentation* or "bear tracks," discussed in the following section. Histologically both conditions appear to be identical.

Solitary CHRPE lesions are usually asymptomatic and dark black and may contain areas of depigmentation (lacunae) within the lesion. The borders of the lesion are sharply defined and often there is a thin halo of depigmentation at the edges of the lesion site. CHRPE lesions are usually 1 to 2 disc diameters in size at the posterior pole and much larger when located in the retinal periphery.

Histologically, there is hyperpigmentation in the region of the CHRPE lesion site and the retinal pigment epithelium cells, although taller, are still only one layer in thickness often containing more pigment granules, which are larger and more globular in shape than the granules within normal retinal pigment epithelium cells nearby. The halo at the edge of the CHRPE lesion is depigmented due to the lack of granules within the retinal pigment epithelium at that site. The overlying neurosensory retina shows degenerative changes, which are probably responsible for the visual field deficits present, otherwise changes in overlying retinal tissues are minimal. Drusen and lipofuscin deposits are rarely seen, and the overlying retinal vessels are usually normal. Visual field deficits can be noted with careful perimetry testing.

Congenital hypertrophy of the retinal pigment epithelium is a unilateral lesion, considered to be benign and stationary with little tendency to grow. If and when these lesions do grow, they do so very slowly. The most important point about CHRPE lesions is that they be recognized for what they really are, and they must be differentiated from choroidal nevi and choroidal melanomas.

Pigmentary Lesions of the Peripheral Retina   **Plate 47**

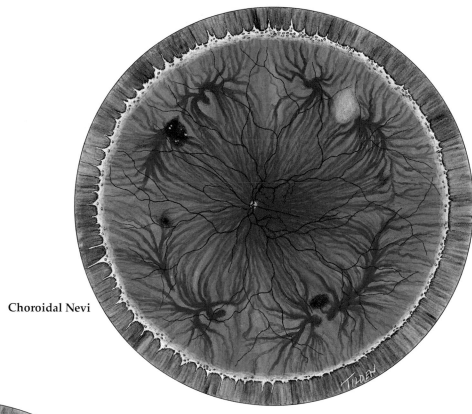

Choroidal Nevi

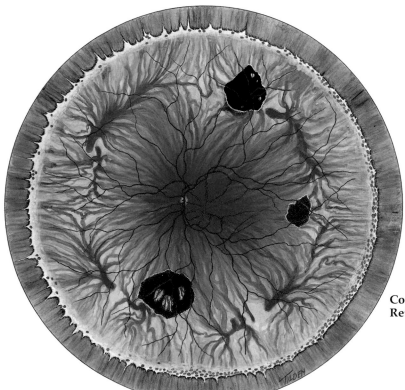

**Congenital Hypertrophy of
Retinal Pigment Epithelium (CHRPE)**

Plate 48   **Congenital Grouped Pigmentation ("Bear Tracks")**

Congenital Grouped Pigmentation ("Bear Tracks")

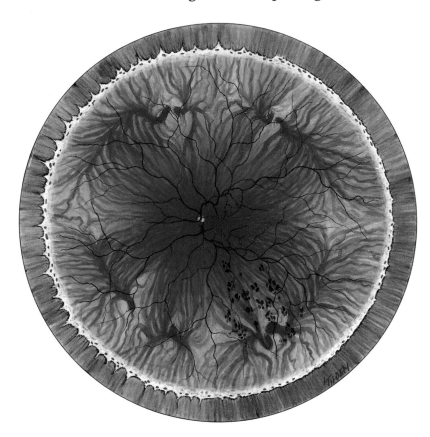

Congenital grouped pigmentation is a series of pigmented plaquelike lesions that are oval in shape and are due to hyperpigmentation of the retinal pigment epithelium (increased numbers of intracellular pigment granules). The overlying retina is normal. The lesions have sharply defined borders and vary in color from brown to black. The lesions occur in clusters, which appear wider as one goes toward the periphery and are usually located in a sector or quadrant of retina. The clustered arrangement of these multifocal lesions resemble paw prints of an animal and therefore have been termed "bear tracks."

The patient is usually asymptomatic, and the lesions are considered benign and identical to the solitary lesions found in congenital hypertrophy of the retinal pigment epithelium (CHRPE). There is no particular sexual predilection. The differential diagnosis of multifocal CHRPE includes retinal pigment dispersion from inflammation or from trauma as well as sector retinitis pigmentosa.

Metastatic Tumors to the Choroid

Tumors that metastasize to the globe usually do so via the bloodstream and often involve some part of the uveal tract. Metastasis directly to the retina are extremely rare. Metastases to the peripheral choroid are less common than to the posterior pole region. Although some studies indicate a slight predilection of uveal metastasis for the left eye, there is in fact no statistically significant left-right predilection demonstrable.

Metastatic tumors to the uveal tract are rare in children and are therefore found, for the most part, in adults. Breast carcinoma is the most frequent tumor to metastasize to the eye, therefore uveal metastases occur more frequently in women. Lung carcinoma is the second most common primary tumor to metastasize to the eye, followed by gastrointestinal tract and kidney carcinomas. Sarcomas rarely metastasize to the globe. On occasion, a skin melanoma may metastasize to the uveal tract (approximately one in two hundred cases).

Ophthalmoscopically, metastatic choroidal tumors can be flat, irregular in shape or, less commonly, dome-shaped, poorly pigmented, or amelanotic. Typically, the lesions are multifocal, multinodular, and often bilateral, especially if the primary tumor is breast carcinoma. In many metastatic tumors, there is a typical geographic distribution of brown pigmentation on the lesion's inner surface. There is also a serous detachment of the retina, which is often greater in size relative to the tumor size than would be found in a primary choroidal melanoma.

Fluorescein angiography, ultrasonography, ^{32}P testing and a comprehensive medical examination in addition to indirect ophthalmoscopy are important in establishing the diagnosis and plan of treatment for the patient. The differential diagnosis of metastatic tumors of the choroid is similar to that listed for choroidal melanomas in Table 10.1 (page 100).

Metastatic Choroidal Tumors   Plate 49

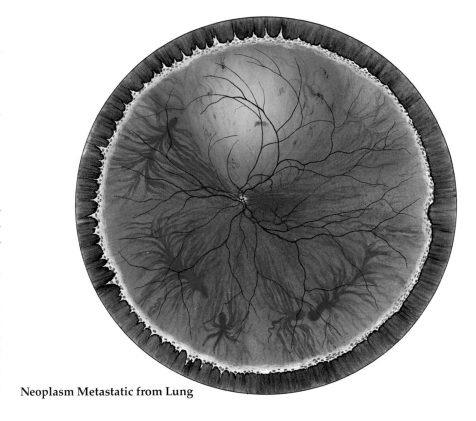

Neoplasm Metastatic from Lung

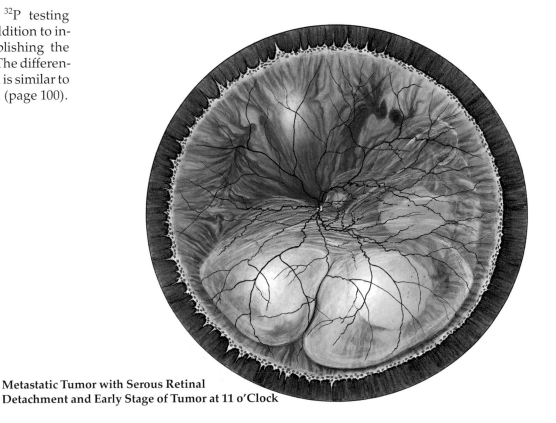

**Metastatic Tumor with Serous Retinal
Detachment and Early Stage of Tumor at 11 o'Clock**

Choroidal Melanomas

Melanomas of the uveal tract are considered to be the most common primary intraocular tumor that affects older adults and is usually diagnosed between the fourth and seventh decades. There is no particular sexual predilection. The melanoma is usually unilateral, and there is no preference for either the left or the right eye. Bilateral cases of melanoma are very rare.

Peripheral choroidal melanomas are asymptomatic when they are small and usually do not interfere with a patient's vision. The lesions are elevated and vary in color from dark brown to grey or even to a creamy yellow (amelanotic). Choroidal melanomas tend to be larger (greater than 5 mm in diameter) than choroidal nevi and are at least 2 mm in height. A localized serous detachment of the retina in and around the melanoma may be present and provide visual symptoms.

Larger choroidal melanomas may break through Bruch's membrane in a mushroom configuration, leading to a serous or exudative retinal detachment. Also, subretinal and intraretinal hemorrhages may occur. In some cases, there is breakthrough bleeding, and a vitreous hemorrhage with sudden visual loss may be the initial findings on examination. That is why ultrasonography should be carried out in adult patients who present with a vitreous hemorrhage in which the media are too cloudy to carry out thorough indirect ophthalmoscopy.

Peripheral choroidal melanomas have poorly defined borders and have several different types of growth patterns. The smaller tumors may be oval, whereas the larger tumors that penetrate Bruch's membrane often have a mushroom shape. The larger tumors often have an associated serous retinal detachment. In some instances, the tumor may actually abut the posterior lens capsule and indent the posterior surface of the lens. The retinal pigment epithelium overlying the choroidal tumor often has pigmentary changes (drusen) and may develop an orange pigment, which has been identified as lipofuscin. Cystoid degeneration of the overlying neurosensory retina is also a common finding.

The Callender classification has defined six categories of melanoma as follows: (1) spindle A, (2) spindle B, (3) fascicular, (4) mixed, (5) necrotic, and (6) epithelioid. Fluorescein angiography, ultrasonography, ^{32}P testing, and a complete medical examination are important modalities in establishing the diagnosis and extent of tumor involvement in a given individual. However, it is not possible, at this time, to tell from these tests and from the ophthalmoscopic appearance of the choroidal melanoma which tissue type one is dealing with, thereby making patient management much more difficult. The differential diagnostic entities to be considered in peripheral uveal melanomas are listed in Table 10.1.

Table 10.1.

Differential Diagnosis of Peripheral Uveal Melanomas

Choroidal nevus

Rhegmatogenous retinal detachment

Choroidal effusion syndrome

Choroidal detachment

Choroidal hemorrhage

Subretinal hemorrhage

Metastatic tumor

Congenital hypertrophy of the retinal pigment epithelium

Choroidal hemangioma

Prehyaloid hemorrhage

Peripheral exudative hemorrhagic chorioretinopathy

Posterior scleritis

Occult intraocular foreign body

Benign reactive lymphoid hyperplasia of the uveal tract

Choroidal Melanomas **Plate 50**

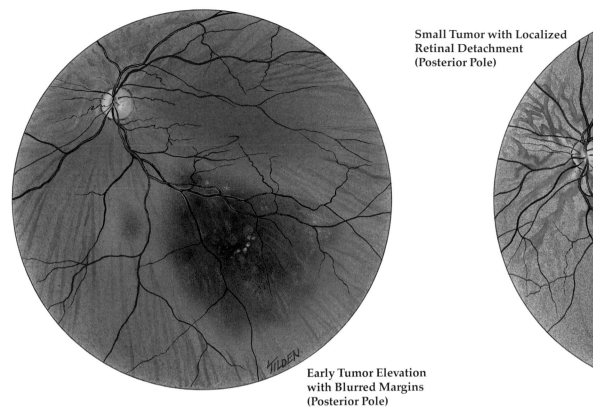

Small Tumor with Localized Retinal Detachment (Posterior Pole)

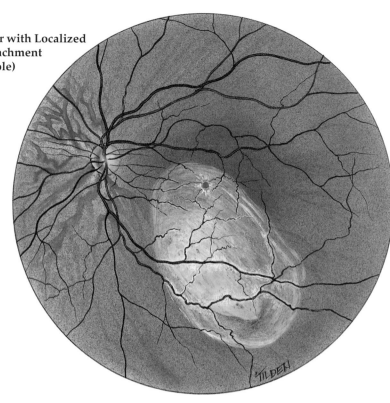

Early Tumor Elevation with Blurred Margins (Posterior Pole)

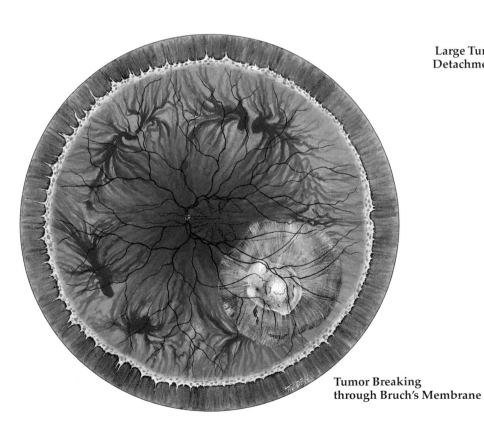

Large Tumor with Serous Detachment of the Retina

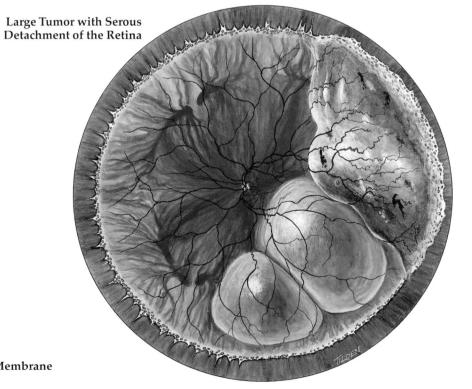

Tumor Breaking through Bruch's Membrane

Retinitis Pigmentosa 11

Retinitis pigmentosa is a progressive primary pigmentary dystrophy of the retina characterized by a collection of bone spicule-shaped pigment located in the midperiphery of the retina, a marked narrowing of the retinal arterioles, night blindness, altered dark adaptation, a diminished electroretinogram, and constricted visual fields (ring scotomas). The retinal veins appear normal in retinitis pigmentosa, as do the optic nerve heads and the maculae initially. However, as the disease progresses, optic pallor (waxy) usually will develop and in some cases cystoid macular edema with macular atrophy also will be present.

There are wide variations in the appearance of the fundus in patients with retinitis pigmentosa. The disease is usually bilateral and involves all four quadrants of the fundus. Cases of unilateral and sector retinitis pigmentosa have been reported. In some cases there is lack of abnormal fundus pigmentation, which has been termed retinitis pigmentosa sine pigments.

Retinitis pigmentosa has autosomal recessive, autosomal dominant, and sex-linked recessive (the most disabling) modes of inheritance and can also be sporadic. The disease usually starts in the first decade of life with the appearance of finely pigmented dots in the midperiphery of the fundus and slowly progresses to the bone-spicule pigment architecture with the development of a ring scotoma. Electroretinogram changes usually precede ophthalmoscopic changes in retinitis pigmentosa.

There is a higher incidence of myopia (75 %), posterior subcapsular lens opacities (up to 60 %), and chronic open-angle glaucoma (3 %) in retinitis pigmentosa patients. In addition to optic atrophy, drusen and hamartomas of the optic nerve head have been noted. Strabismus, progressive external ophthalmoplegia, keratoconus, and microphthalmos have been found in related syndromes.

With increasing age, there is progressive opacification and degeneration of the vitreous. Increased pigment deposits have been observed of the vitreous. Retinal tears and detachments are infrequent in retinitis pigmentosa patients.

There are a number of disorders that comprise the differential diagnosis of retinitis pigmentosa. These are listed in Table 11.1.

Table 11.1.

Differential Diagnosis of Retinitis Pigmentosa

Laurence-Moon syndrome
Bardet-Biedl syndrome
Bassen-Kornzweig syndrome
Refsum's syndrome
Usher's syndrome
Friedreich's ataxia
Goldmann-Favre disease
Hallgren's syndrome
Cockayne's syndrome
Pelizaeus-Merzbacher syndrome
Mucopolysaccharidoses
   Type I   (Hurler's syndrome)
   Type II (Hunter's syndrome)
   Type III (Sanfilippo's syndrome)
   Type IV (Morquio's syndrome)
Congenital rubella
Syphilis
Cystinosis
Myotonic dystrophy
Neuronal ceroid lipofuscinosis
Trauma
Turner's syndrome
Lignac-Fanconi syndrome
Leber's congenital amaurosis
Kearns-Sayre syndrome
Drug toxicities
   Phenothiazines
   Chloroquine
   Vitamin A

Retinitis Pigmentosa   **Plate 51**

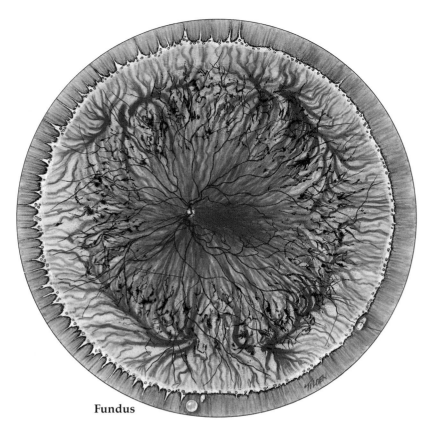

Fundus

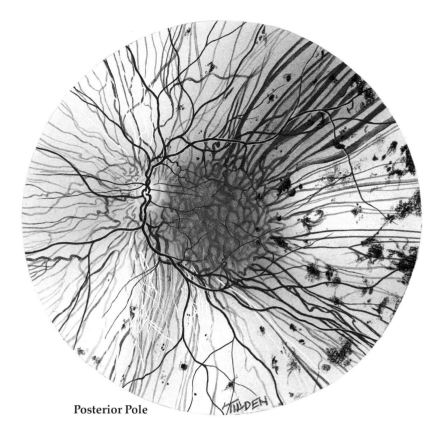

Posterior Pole

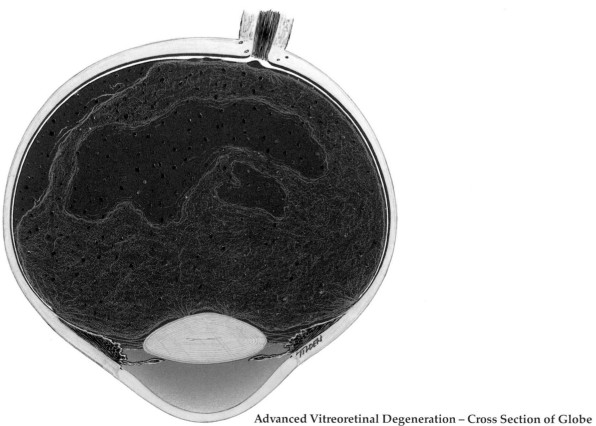

Advanced Vitreoretinal Degeneration – Cross Section of Globe

Plate 51   **Retinitis Pigmentosa**

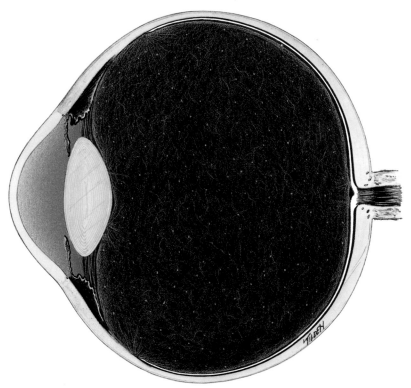

Progressive Vitreoretinal Degeneration – Stage I

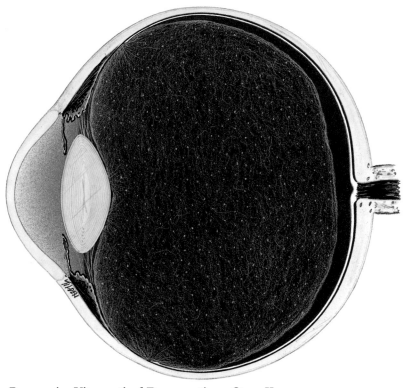

Progressive Vitreoretinal Degeneration – Stage II

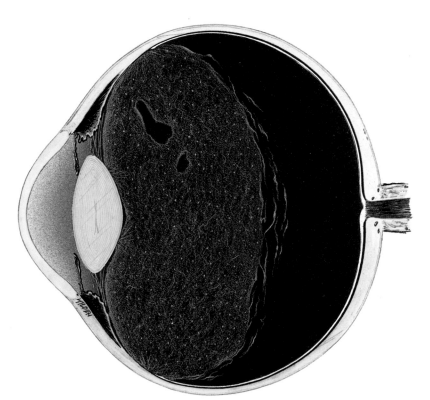

Progressive Vitreoretinal Degeneration – Stage III

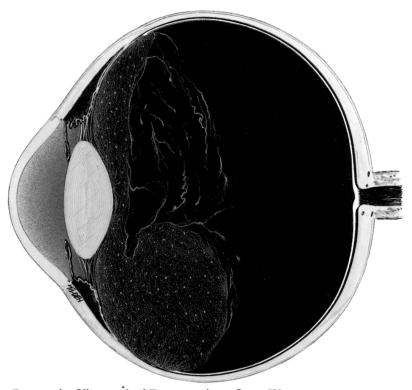

Progressive Vitreoretinal Degeneration – Stage IV

Developmental Disorders: Colobomas of the Retina and Choroid

Plate 52   **Coloboma of the Retina and Choroid**

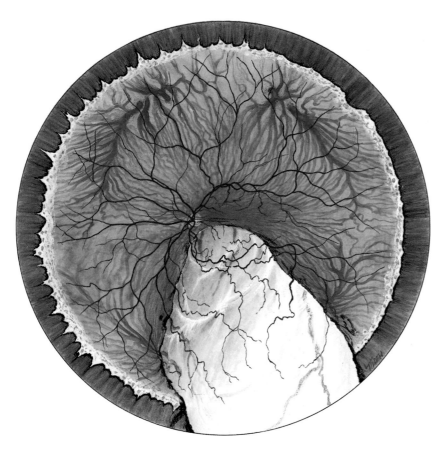

Colobomas of the retina and choroid (0.14 % incidence) represent a developmental abnormality usually involving the closure of the fetal fissure during embryonic development. Colobmas can involve the optic nervehead, retina, choroid, ciliary body, lens, and iris tissue. The mechanism of coloboma formation is still not well understood, but has been associated, in some cases, with chromosomal defects such as trisomy 13 and trisomy 18, as well as with use of toxic drugs such as thalidomide.

Ophthalmoscopically, the coloboma region apears to be almost devoid of retinal and choroidal tissues, making the subjacent sclera easily visible. There is a rudimentary membrane containing retinal tissue and vessels that may cover the inner surface of some colobomas. At the edges of a coloboma there is often a highly pigmented border.

Colobomas tend to be bilateral (50 % of cases) and typical colobomas are usually in the inferonasal quadrant. Atypical colobomas may be present in the superior quadrants. No specific hereditary patterns have been established for colobomas in general, but there are reports of sporadic cases as well as autosomal dominant and autosomal recessive transmission.

Colobomas may give rise to retinal detachments in 40 % of cases. The retinal break may lie within the colobomatous (depigmented) area, making its visualization extremely difficult. Scleral buckling surgery is used to treat retinal detachments in eyes with colobomas of the retina and choroid, but the visual prognosis in these cases is poor compared to the patient with routine rhegmatogenous retinal detachment.

Long-Standing Retinal Detachments   13

Intraocular Fibrosis
Demarcation Lines

Long-standing retinal detachments often have a variety of characteristic structural changes, for example, demarcation lines, macrocysts, and subretinal bands, which are discussed in this chapter.

Intraocular Fibrosis

Intraocular fibrosis may be found in acute as well as chronic cases of retinal detachment and is due to abnormal cellular proliferation in the vitreous gel and the neurosensory retina. Abnormal membranes may also be found on the preretinal and subretinal surfaces of the neurosensory retina. Intraocular fibrosis may also take place within the neurosensory retina in such conditions as star folds and macular pucker.

The cellular origins of abnormal vitreoretinal membranes are listed in Table 13.1. In most cases, the membranes are derived from either the Müller (glial) cells or the retinal pigment epithelium.

Abnormal cellular proliferation leads to membrane formation, which may, in turn, undergo a contraction process, leading to folds in the retina, localized traction, and/or rhegmatogenous retinal detachments. Extramacular retinal folds are termed *star folds*; abnormal folds within the macula are termed *macular pucker*.

In some cases, there is a relentless progression of these membranes, leading to *proliferative vitreoretinopathy (PVR)* or *massive periretinal proliferation (MPP)*, wherein the entire retina is thrown into a large funnel-shaped star fold whose apex is at the optic nerve head. In these cases, there is extensive liquefaction or syneresis of the vitreous gel posteriorly with an increased condensation of the anterior vitreous gel (at the base of the funnel). A simple classification of proliferative vitreoretinopathy is outlined in Table 13.2.

Table 13.1.

Cellular Sources of Vitreoretinal Membranes

Whole blood
  Lymphocytes
  Leukocytes
  Monocytes
  Platelets

Vascular endothelium

Ciliary body (nonpigmented epithelium)

Fibroblasts

Hyalocytes

Retinal pigment epithelium (fibroblastic transformation)

Müller cells (glial)

Table 13.2.

The Classification of Retinal Detachment with Proliferative Vitreoretinopathy (PVR)

Grade	Name	Clinical Signs
A	Minimal	Vitreous haze, vitreous pigment clumps
B	Moderate	Wrinkling of the inner retinal surface, rolled edge of retinal break, retinal stiffness, vessel tortuosity
C	Marked	Full thickness fixed retinal folds
C-1		One quadrant
C-2		Two quadrants
C-3		Three quadrants
D	Massive	Fixed retinal folds in four quadrants
D-1		Wide funnel shape
D-2		Narrow funnel shape*
D-3		Closed funnel (optic nervehead not visible)

* Narrow funnel shape exists when the anterior end of the funnel can be seen by indirect ophthalmoscopy within the 45° field of a +20D condensing lens (Nikon or equivalent).
Reprinted with permission from The Retina Society Terminology Committee: The classification of retinal detachment with proliferative vitreoretinopathy. Ophthalmology 90 (2): 121–5. Philadelphia, Lippincott/Harper & Row, 1983

Proliferative Vitreoretinopathy (PVR)   **Plate 53**

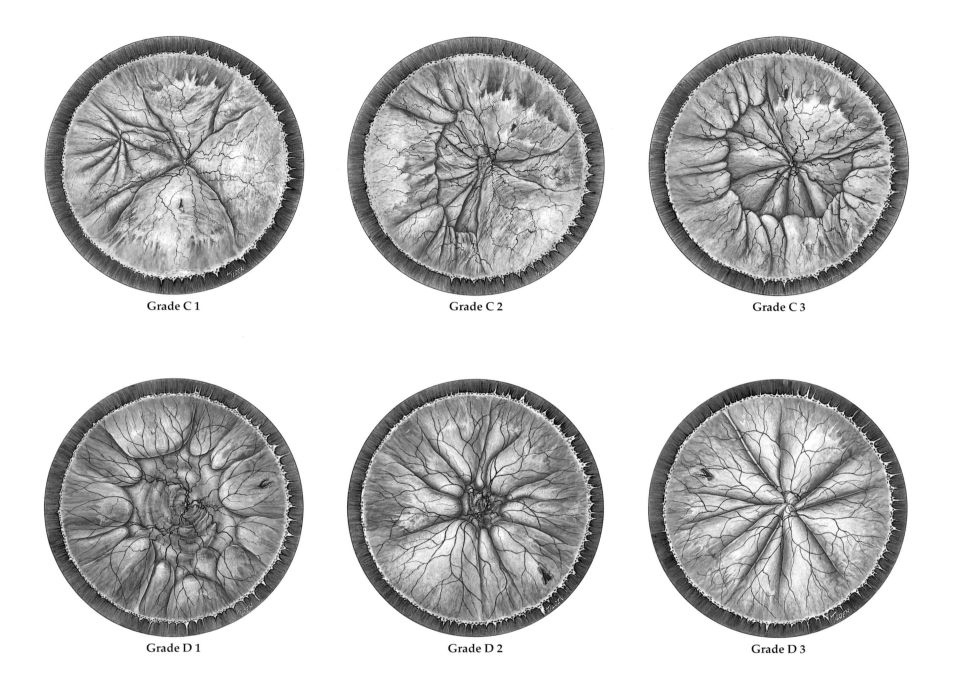

Grade C 1   Grade C 2   Grade C 3

Grade D 1   Grade D 2   Grade D 3

Intraocular fibrosis can lead to a variety of intraocular membranes in the posterior segment of the globe, and their classification is outlined in Table 13.3.

In chronic retinal detachments, there are proliferative and degenerative retinal pigment epithelium changes, including increased pigmentary material in the subretinal fluid, and, in some cases, nonpigmented subretinal strands of tissue are present that act as a hammock supporting overlying detached neurosensory retinal tissue. The ends of these subretinal strands are attached to either the retinal pigment epithelium or to the subretinal surface of the neurosensory retina.

Chronically detached retina tends to be thinner and more transparent than freshly detached retina. The subretinal fluid may be more viscous, and, in cases of tiny retinal breaks, one may see shifting subretinal fluid, which is not seen in fresh rhegmatogenous retinal detachments. Fixed retinal folds and a more rigid detached retina are commonly noted in long-standing retinal detachments. Microcystoid spaces, usually at the level of the outer plexiform and inner nuclear layers, are found in chronically detached retinas. These cystic changes are reversible if the retina is reattached within a reasonable period of time.

In chronic retinal detachments, retinal tear flaps and opercula have an opportunity to degenerate and shrink so that their size is much smaller than the aperture size of the tear site. In contrast, opercula and retinal tear flaps in fresh retinal tears usually are the same size as the retinal tear aperture.

Large *intraretinal macrocysts* can develop in a period of several months to years in a long-standing retinal detachment. These macrocysts are commonly found in inferior retinal detachments due to such conditions as an inferior temporal dialysis of the young. Intraretinal macrocysts are often elevated and protrude into the subretinal space and are found mostly near the equator and only rarely at the posterior pole. The cysts collapse and regress rapidly after surgical reattachment of the retina and do not require direct drainage of the cystic cavity itself.

Table 13.3.

Classification of Intraocular Membranes in the Posterior Segment of the Eye

Lens capsule (remnants) membranes

Cyclitic membranes

Vitreoretinal membranes
  Anteroposterior traction
    Truncated cone membranes
    Stalk membranes
      Optic nerve head
      Retina
  Equatorial traction
    Equatorial membranes
    Bridging membranes
  Epiretinal traction
    Macular pucker
    Extramacular pucker
    Star fold

Intraretinal membranes
  Tangential traction
    Macular pucker
    Extramacular pucker
    Star fold

Subretinal membranes
  Tangential traction
    Clothesline
    Placoid
      Fishnet
      Discoid
    Napkin ring (peripapillary)
  Anteroposterior traction
    Clothesline
    Placoid
      Fishnet
    Napkin ring

Demarcation Lines

Demarcation lines are found in slowly progressive or chronic retinal detachments. In these cases, the amount of subretinal fluid may stabilize for some time. The presence of the subretinal fluid induces an irritation or friction as it moves back and forth, leading to secondary proliferative changes of the retinal pigment epithelium at the boundary line between the attached and detached retina. Fibrous metaplasia of the retinal pigment epithelium may also occur.

Ultimately a hyperpigmented line or, in some cases, a hypopigmented line develops that is termed the demarcation (friction) line. The demarcation line often, but not always, serves as a barrier to the further progression of the retinal detachment. In some eyes, several concentric demarcation lines are present, similiar to high-water marks, indicating several waves of activity or progression of the retinal detachment interspersed with periods of nonprogression or stability. Often demarcation lines form a partial circle and within that circle one usually finds the causative retinal break.

The characteristics of long-standing retinal detachments are outlined in Table 13.4.

Table 13.4.

Characteristics of Long-Standing Retinal Detachments

Detached retina
  Shrinkage of retinal tear flaps and opercula
  Thinning and atrophy (↑ transparency of retina)
  Microcystoid degeneration
  Intraretinal macrocysts
  Fixed folds (PVR)
    ↓ Mobility of retina (↑ rigidity)
  Subretinal fluid
    ↑ Viscosity (↑ protein)
  Pigment debris
  Shifting subretinal fluid (with very small retinal holes)

Retinal pigment epithelium
  Hyperpigmentation
  Hypopigmentation and atrophy
  Fibrous metaplasia
  Fibroplastic transformation (MPP)
  Demarcation line formation

Intraocular fibrosis
  Vitreal membranes
  Preretinal membranes
  Intraneurosensory membranes
    Star folds
    Macular pucker
  Subretinal strands (nonpigmented)
  Proliferative vitreoretinopathy (PVR)

Long-Standing Retinal Detachment with Demarcation Line, Intraretinal Macrocysts and Fixed Retinal Folds   **Plate 54**

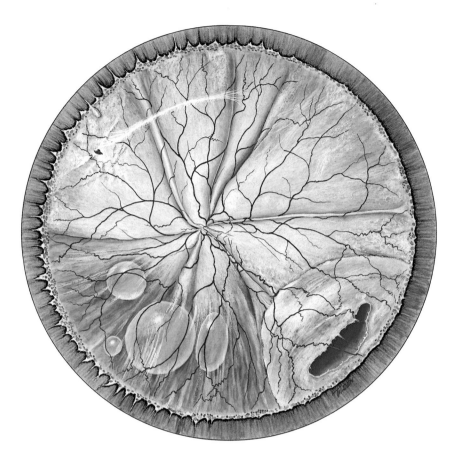

Fundus Color Code   14

Many years ago, Dr. Charles Schepens devised a system of sketching the fundus as a way of recording the findings on indirect ophthalmoscopy with scleral depression. This technique has served as an invaluable aid in improving our comprehension and overall understanding of retinal diseases as well as planning vitreoretinal surgery in specific patients.

As a by-product of the fundus sketching system a universal color code was developed to help standardize and interpret fundus drawings. The fundus code is outlined in Table 14.1. In its simplest form, the fundus color code is organized along the following lines:

Red: attached retina, retinal arterioles, fresh hemorrhage, vortex veins, retinal tears and holes;

Blue: retinal veins, detached retina, outline of the ora serrata, cystoid degeneration;

Green: any opacities in the eye, vitreous hemorrhage, cotton wool patches, vitreous membranes, and intraocular foreign bodies;

Brown: uveal tissue, pars plana cysts, pigment beneath detached retina, choroidal tumors, and choroidal detachments;

Yellow: retinal exudates, intraretinal edema, drusen, post-photocoagulation burns (edema) of the retina;

Black: pigment in choroid, outline of the long and short posterior ciliary vessels and nerves, pigmented demarcation lines at edge of long-standing retinal detachment, pigmented laser photocoagulation scars.

A more comprehensive and detailed description of the fundus color code is provided in Table 14.1. In the pages following the table, the entire fundus color code is illustrated. For each feature listed in Table 14.1 the ophthalmologist's sketch representation is shown side-by-side with a fundus painting of the condition as viewed through the ophthalmoscope.

Table 14.1 Fundus Color Code[1]

Code[2]	Fundus Color and Characteristics	Code[2]	Fundus Color and Characteristics	Code[2]	Fundus Color and Characteristics
[R]	**Red** *Solid*	**[B]**	**Blue** *Solid*	**[Br]**	**Brown** *Solid*
1	Retinal arterioles	15	Detached retina	46	Uveal tissue
2	Neovascularization	16	Retinal veins	47	Pars plana cysts
3	Vascular abnormalities or anomalies	17	Outlines of retinal breaks (tears, holes)	48	Ciliary processes (pars plicata)
4	Vortex veins	18	Outline of ora serrata (dentate processes, ora bays)	49	Striae ciliaris
5	Attached retina			50	Pigment beneath detached retina
6	Hemorrhages (preretinal, intraretinal)	19, 20, 21, 22	Meridional [19], radial [20], fixed [21], and circumferential [22] folds	51	Outline of chorioretinal atrophy beneath detached retina
7	Open interior of conventional retinal breaks (tears, holes)	23	Vitreoretinal traction tufts	52	Subretinal, fibrous demarcation lines
8	Open interior of outer layer holes in retinoschisis	24	Retinal granular tags and tufts (cystic, noncystic)	53	Outline of posterior staphyloma
9	Normal macula – drawn as a red dot	25	Outline of flat neovascularization	54	Malignant choroidal melanomas
		26	Outline of lattice degeneration	55	Edge of buckle beneath detached retina
	Crosslined	27	Outline of thin areas of retina	56	Choroidal detachment
10, 11	Open portion of giant tears [10] or large dialyses [11]	28	Intraretinal cysts (with overlying curvilinear stripes to show configuration)		
12	Inner portion of chorioretinal atrophy		*Crosslined*	**[Y]**	**Yellow** *Solid*
13	Open portion of retinal holes in inner layer of retinoschisis	29	Inner layer of retinoschisis	57	Intraretinal edema
14	Inner portion of thin areas of retina	30	White-with- or -without-pressure (label)	58	Intra- or subretinal hard yellow exudate
		31	Detached pars plana epithelium anterior to separation of ora serrata	59	Deposits in retinal pigmented epithelium
		32	Rolled edges of retinal tears (curved lines)	60	Detached maculae in some retinal separations
				61	Postphotocoagulation retinal edema
			Stippled or circled	62	Substance of long and short posterior ciliary nerves
		33	Cystoid degeneration		
					Stippled or dotted
			Interrupted lines	63	Drusen
		34	Outline of change in area or folds of detached retina because of shifting fluid		
				[Bl]	**Black** *Solid*
				64, 65, 66	Pigment within detached retina (lattice [64], flap of horseshoe tear [65], paravascular pigment [66])
		[G]	**Green** *Solid*	67, 68	Pigment in choroid [67] or pigmented epithelial hyperpigmentation in areas of detached retina [68]
		35	Opacities in the media (cornea, anterior chamber, lens, vitreous); label specifically	69	Pigmented demarcation lines at attached margin of detached retina or within detached retina
		36	Vitreous hemorrhage	70	Nevi
		37	Vitreous membranes	71, 72	Sheathed vessels outlined or solid black, depending upon extent (lattice [71], retinoschisis [72])
		38	Hyaloid ring	73	Edge of buckle beneath attached retina
		39	Intraocular foreign bodies	74	Outline of long posterior ciliary vessels and nerves (pigmented)
		40	Retinal operculum	75	Outline of short ciliary vessels and nerves
		41	Cotton-wool patches	76	Outline of chorioretinal atrophy
		42	Pearls at the ora serrata	77	Hyperpigmentation as a result of previous treatment with cryotherapy, photocoagulation, or diathermy
		43	Outline of elevated neovascularization		
			Stippled or dotted		
		44	Asteroid hyalosis		
		45	Frosting or snowflakes on cystoid, retinoschisis, or lattice degeneration		

[1] From Morse P: Vitreoretinal Disease. A Manual for Diagnosis and Treatment. Chicago, Year Book Medical Publishers Inc., 1979. Tables 2-1 through 2-6. pp. 41–44.

[2] The numbers given in these columns refer to the specific figures illustrating that feature in the illustrated fundus color code that follows this table.

Fundus Color Code

Color	Feature	Ophthalmologist's Sketch Representation	Ophthalmoscopic Finding	Color Code Number (See Table 14.1)
Red *Solid*	Retinal arterioles			1
	Neovascularization			2
	Vascular abnormalities or anomalies			3
	Vortex veins			4
	Attached retina			5
	Hemorrhages (preretinal, intraretinal)			6

Fundus Color Code

Color	Feature	Ophthalmologist's Sketch Representation	Ophthalmoscopic Finding	Color Code Number (See Table 14.1)
Red *Solid*	Open interior of conventional retinal breaks (tears, holes)			7
	Open interior of outer layer holes in retinoschisis			8
	Normal macula-drawn as a red dot			9
Red *Crosslined*	Open portion of giant tears			10
	Open portion of large dialyses			11
	Inner portion of chorioretinal atrophy			12

Fundus Color Code

Color	Feature	Ophthalmologist's Sketch Representation	Ophthalmoscopic Finding	Color Code Number (See Table 14.1)
Red *Crosslined*	Open portion of retinal holes in inner layer of retinoschisis			13
	Inner portion of thin areas of retina			14
Blue *Solid*	Detached retina			15
	Retinal veins			16
	Outlines of retinal breaks (tears, holes)			17
	Outline of ora serrata (dentate processes, ora bays)			18

Fundus Color Code

Color	Feature	Ophthalmologist's Sketch Representation	Ophthalmoscopic Finding	Color Code Number (See Table 14.1)
Blue *Solid*	Meridional folds			19
	Radial folds			20
	Fixed folds			21
	Circumferential folds			22
	Vitreoretinal traction tufts			23
	Retinal granular tags and tufts (cystic, noncystic)			24

Fundus Color Code

Color	Feature	Ophthalmologist's Sketch Representation	Ophthalmoscopic Finding	Color Code Number (See Table 14.1)
Blue *Solid*	Outline of flat neovascularization			25
	Outline of lattice degeneration			26
	Outline of thin areas of retina			27
	Intraretinal cysts (with overlying curvilinear stripes to show configuration)	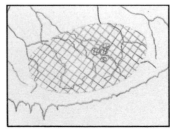	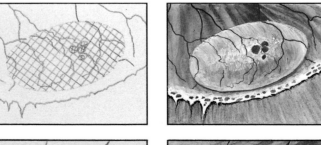	28
Blue *Crosslined*	Inner layer of retinoschisis			29
	White-with- or -without-pressure (label)		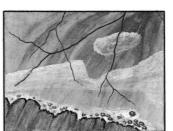	30

Fundus Color Code

Color	Feature	Ophthalmologist's Sketch Representation	Ophthalmoscopic Finding	Color Code Number (See Table 14.1)
Blue *Crosslined*	Detached pars plana epithelium anterior to separation of ora serrata			31
	Rolled edges of retinal tears (curved lines)			32
Blue *Stippled or circled*	Cystoid degeneration			33
Blue *Interrupted lines*	Outline of change in area or folds of detached retina because of shifting fluid			34
Green *Solid*	Opacities in the media (cornea, anterior chamber, lens, vitreous); label specifically			35
	Vitreous hemorrhage			36

Fundus Color Code

Color	Feature	Ophthalmologist's Sketch Representation	Ophthalmoscopic Finding	Color Code Number (See Table 14.1)
Green *Solid*	Vitreous membranes			37
	Hyaloid ring			38
	Intraocular foreign bodies			39
	Retinal operculum			40
	Cotton-wool patches			41
	Pearls at the ora serrata			42

Fundus Color Code

Color	Feature	Ophthalmologist's Sketch Representation	Ophthalmoscopic Finding	Color Code Number (See Table 14.1)
Green *Solid*	Outline of elevated neovascularization			43
Green *Stippled or dotted*	Asteroid hyalosis			44
	Frosting or snowflakes on cystoid, retinoschisis, or lattice degeneration			45
Brown *Solid*	Uveal tissue			46
	Pars plana cysts			47
	Ciliary processes (pars plicata)			48

Fundus Color Code

Color	Feature	Ophthalmologist's Sketch Representation	Ophthalmoscopic Finding	Color Code Number (See Table 14.1)
Brown *Solid*	Striae ciliaris			49
	Pigment beneath detached retina			50
	Outline of chorioretinal atrophy beneath detached retina			51
	Subretinal, fibrous demarcation lines			52
	Outline of posterior staphyloma			53
	Malignant choroidal melanomas			54

Fundus Color Code

Color	Feature	Ophthalmologist's Sketch Representation	Ophthalmoscopic Finding	Color Code Number (See Table 14.1)
Brown *Solid*	Edge of buckle beneath detached retina			55
	Choroidal detachment			56
Yellow *Solid*	Intraretinal edema			57
	Intra- or subretinal hard yellow exudate			58
	Deposits in retinal pigmented epithelium			59
	Detached maculae in some retinal separations			60

Fundus Color Code

Color	Feature	Ophthalmologist's Sketch Representation	Ophthalmoscopic Finding	Color Code Number (See Table 14.1)
Yellow *Solid*	Postphotocoagulation retinal edema			**61**
	Substance of long and short posterior ciliary nerves			**62**
Yellow *Stippled or dotted*	Drusen			**63**
Black *Solid*	Pigment within detached retina (lattice)			**64**
	Pigment within detached retina (flap of horseshoe tear)			**65**
	Pigment within detached retina (paravascular pigment)			**66**

Fundus Color Code

Color	Feature	Ophthalmologist's Sketch Representation	Ophthalmoscopic Finding	Color Code Number (See Table 14.1)
Black *Solid*	Pigment in choroid			67
	Pigmented epithelial hyperpigmentation in areas of detached retina			68
	Pigmented demarcation lines at attached margin of detached retina or within detached retina			69
	Nevi			70
	Sheathed vessels outlined or solid black, depending upon extent (lattice)			71
	Sheathed vessels outlined or solid black, depending upon extent (retinoschisis)			72

Fundus Color Code

Color	Feature	Ophthalmologist's Sketch Representation	Ophthalmoscopic Finding	Color Code Number (See Table 14.1)
Black *Solid*	Edge of buckle beneath attached retina			73
	Outline of long posterior ciliary vessels and nerves (pigmented)			74
	Outline of short ciliary vessels and nerves			75
	Outline of chorioretinal atrophy			76
	Hyperpigmentation as a result of previous treatment with cryotherapy, photocoagulation or diathermy			77

Bibliographies and References

General Bibliography

Apple DJ, Raab MF: Clinicopathologic Correlation of Ocular Disease. A Text and Stereoscopic Atlas, 2nd ed. St. Louis, Mosby, 1978. 526 pp

Bell FC, Stenstrom WS: Atlas of the Peripheral Retina. Philadelphia, Saunders, 1983. 232 pp

Benson WE: Retinal Detachment. Diagnosis and Management. Hagerstown, MD, Harper & Row, 1980. 196 pp

Byer NE: The Peripheral Retina in Profile. A Stereoscopic Atlas. Torrence, CA, Criterion Press, 1982. 159 pp

Chignell AH: Retinal Detachment Surgery. New York, Springer-Verlag, 1980. 166 pp

Curtin BJ: The Myopias: Basic Science and Clinical Management. Philadelphia, Harper & Row, 1985. 495 pp

Freeman H, Hirose T, Schepens CL: Vitreous Surgery and Advances in Fundus Diagnosis and Treatment. New York, Appleton-Century-Crofts, 1977. 681 pp

Kanski JJ: Retinal Detachment: A Colour Manual of Diagnosis and Treatment. London, Butterworth, 1986. 161 pp

Krill A: Krill's Hereditary Retinal and Choroidal Diseases, vol 1, 2. Hagerstown, MD, Harper & Row, 1977. 1371 pp

L'Esperance Jr FA, James Jr WA: Diabetic Retinopathy. Clinical Evaluation and Management. St. Louis, Mosby, 1981. 294 pp

McPherson A (ed): New and Controversial Aspects of Vitreoretinal Surgery. St. Louis, Mosby, 1977. 455 pp

Morse P: Vitreoretinal Disease. A Manual for Diagnosis and Treatment. Chicago, Year Book Medical Publishers, 1979. 625 pp

O'Malley C, O'Malley P: The Peripheral Fundus of the Eye. New York, Medcom, 1973. 34 pp

Pruett RC, Regan CD: Retinal Congress. New York, Appleton-Century-Crofts, 1972. 730 pp

Ryan SJ, Dawson AK, Little HL (eds): Retinal Diseases. Orlando, FL, Grune & Stratton, 1985. 282 pp

Schepens CL: Retinal Detachment and Allied Diseases, vols 1, 2. Philadelphia, Saunders, 1983. 1155 pp

Sigelman J: Retinal Diseases: Pathogenesis, Laser Therapy and Surgery. Boston, Little, Brown, 1984. 442 pp

Tasman W, Shields JA: Disorders of the Peripheral Fundus. Hagerstown, MD, Harper & Row, 1980. 227 pp

Tolentino FI, Schepens CL, Freeman HM: Vitreoretinal Disorders. Diagnosis and Management. Philadelphia, Saunders, 1976. 659 pp

Transactions of the New Orleans Academy of Ophthalmology. Symposium on Retina and Retinal Surgery. St. Louis, Mosby, 1969. 406 pp

Transactions of the New Orleans Academy of Ophthalmology. Symposium on Retinal Diseases. St. Louis, Mosby, 1977. 354 pp

Wise GN, Dollery CT, Henkind P: The Retinal Circulation. New York, Harper & Row, 1971. 566 pp

Specific Bibliography

Anatomic Considerations

Allen RA, Miller DH, Straatsma BR: Cysts of the posterior ciliary body (pars plana). Arch Ophthalmol 66: 302–13, 1961

Balazs EA: Molecular morphology of the vitreous body. In Smelser GK (ed): The Structure of the Eye. New York, Academic Press, 1961, pp 293–310

Foos RY: Vitreoretinal juncture, topographical variations. Invest Ophthalmol 11:801–08, 1972

Grignolo A: Fibrous components of the vitreous body. Arch Ophthalmol 47:760–74, 1952

Grignolo A, Schepens CL, Heath P: Cysts of the pars plana ciliaris. Arch Ophthalmol 58:530–45, 1957

Hamilton AM, Taylor W: Significance of pigment granules in the vitreous. Br J Ophthalmol 56:700–02, 1972

Hogan MJ, Alvarado JA, Weddell JE: Histology of the Human Eye. Philadelphia, Saunders, 1971

Johnson BL, Storey JD: Proteinaceous cysts of the ciliary epithelium. I. Their clear nature and immunoelectrophoretic analysis in a case of multiple myeloma. II. Their occurrence in non-myelomatous hypergammaglobulinemic conditions. Arch Ophthalmol 84:166–75, 1970

Marchesani O, Sautter H: Atlas of the Ocular Fundus. [Å. Phillipp, transl.]. New York, Hafner, 1959, pp 1–26

Michaelson IC: Textbook of the Fundus of the Eye, 3rd ed. Edinburgh, Churchill Livingstone, 1980. 910 pp

Okun E: Gross and microscopic pathology in autopsy eyes. I. Introduction and long posterior ciliary nerves. Am J Ophthalmol 50:424–9, 1960

Okun E: Gross and microscopic pathology in autopsy eyes. IV. Pars plana cysts. Am J Ophthalmol 51: 1221–8, 1961

Polyak SL: The Retina. Chicago, University of Chicago Press, 1941. 607 pp

Ruiz RS: Giant cysts of the pars plana. Am J Ophthalmol 72:481–2, 1971

Rutnin U: Fundus appearance in normal eyes. I. The choroid. Am J Ophthalmol 64:821–39, 1967

Rutnin U, Schepens CL: Fundus appearance in normal eyes. II. The standard peripheral fundus and development variations. Am J Ophthalmol 64:840–52, 1967

Rutnin U, Schepens CL: Fundus appearance in normal eyes. III. Peripheral degenerations. Am j Ophthalmol 64:1040–62, 1967

Rutnin U, Schepens CL: Fundus appearance in normal eyes. IV. Retinal breaks and other findings. Am J Ophthalmol 64:1063–78, 1967

Salzmann M: The Anatomy and History of the Human Eyeball in the Normal State: Its Development and Senescence. [EVL Brown, transl.]. Chicago, University of Chicago Press, 1912

Schepens CL: Clinical aspects of pathologic changes in the vitreous body. Am J Ophthalmol 38(1, pt II):8–21, 1954

Schepens CL: Retinal Detachment and Allied Diseases, vol 1. Philadelphia, Saunders, pp 23–36, 134–61, 1983

Shafer DM: Binocular indirect ophthalmoscopy (chapter 2); General discussion: Significance of white-with-pressure. In Schepens CL, Regan CDJ (eds): Controversial Aspects of the Management of Retinal Detachment. Boston, Little, Brown, 1965, p 51

Spencer LM, Foos RY: Paravascular vitreoretinal attachments: Role in retinal tears. Arch Ophthalmol 84:557–64, 1970

Spencer LM, Foos RY, Straatsma BM: Meridional folds, meridional complexes, and associated abnormalities of the peripheral retina. Am J Ophthalmol 70:697–714, 1970

Spencer LM, Foos RY, Straatsma BR: Enclosed bays of the ora serrata: relationship to retinal tears. Arch Ophthalmol 83:421–5, 1970

Straatsma BR, Foos RY, Spender LM: The retina-topography and clinical correlations. In New Orleans Academy of

Ophthalmology: Symposium on the Retina and Retinal Surgery. St. Louis, Mosby, 1969, pp 1–26

Straatsma BR, Hall MV, Allen RA, Crescitelli F: The Retina. Los Angeles, University of California Press, 1969

Straatsma BR, Landers MB, Kreiger AE: The ora serrata in the adult human eye. Arch Ophthalmol 80:3–20, 1968

Straatsma BR, Landers MB, Kreiger AE, Apt L: Topography of the Adult Human Retina. In Straatsma BR, Hall MO, Allen RA, Crescitelli F (eds): The Retina. Morphology, Function and Clinical Characteristics. Berkeley, University of California Press, 1969, pp 379–410

Swann DA: The structure and function of the vitreous. In Pruett RC, Regan CDJ (eds): Retina Congress. New York, Appleton-Century-Crofts, 1974, pp 203–14

Swann DA, Constable IJ: Vitreous structure: II. Role of hyaluronate. Invest Ophthalmol 11:164–8, 1972

Tasman W, Shields JA: Disorders of the Peripheral Fundus. Hagerstown, MD, Harper & Row, 1980

Teng CC, Katzin KM: An anatomic study of the retina, Part I. Nonpigmented epithelium cell proliferation and hole formation. Am J Ophthalmol 34:1237–40, 1951

Thiel HL: Beitrage zur Anatomie der Ora serrata. Ber Dtsch Ophthalmol Ges 58:249–56, 1953

Thiel HL: Zur topographischen und histologischen Situation der Ora serrata. Graefes Arch Ophthalmol 156:590–629, 1955

Thiel R: Atlas of Diseases of the Eye, vol 2. [D Guerry, WJ Geeraets, H Wiesinger, transl.]. Amsterdam, Elsevier, 1963

Tolentino FJ, Schepens CL, Freeman HM: Vitreoretinal Disorders: Diagnosis and Management. Philadelphia, Saunders, 1976. 659 pp

Wolff E: Anatomy of the Eye and Orbit, 6th ed. (revised by R Warwick). Philadelphia, Saunders, 1977. 529 pp

Classification System of Peripheral Retinal Degeneration

Foos RY, Spencer LM, Straatsma BR: Trophic degenerations of the peripheral retina. In New Orleans Academy of Ophthalmology: Symposium on the Retina and Retinal Surgery. St. Louis, Mosby, 1969, pp 90–102

Spencer LM, Straatsma BR, Foos RY: Tractional degenerations of the peripheral retina. In New Orleans Academy of Ophthalmology: Symposium on the Retina and Retinal Surgery. St. Louis, Mosby, 1969, pp 103–27

Straatsma BR, Foos RY: Part II. Peripheral retinal disorders. Classification. In L'Esperance Jr FA (ed): Current Diagnosis and Management of Chorioretinal Diseases. St. Louis, Mosby, 1977, pp 97–118

Developmental Variations of the Peripheral Fundus

Ora Serrata Bays

Maggiore L: L'ora serrata nell'occhio umano. (Morfologia, sviluppo anatomia comparata e fisiologia). Ann Oftalmol Clin Ocul 52:625–723, 1924

Rutnin U, Schepens, CL: Fundus appearance in normal eyes II. The standard peripheral fundus and developmental variations. Am J Ophthalmol 64:840–52, 1967

Schepens CL: The standard peripheral fundus and its variations, In Schepens CL: Retinal Detachment and Allied Diseases, vol 1. Philadelphia, Saunders, 1983, pp 134–61

Spencer LM, Foos RY, Straatsma BR: Enclosed bays of the ora serrata. Arch Ophthalmol 83:421–5, 1970

Straatsma BR, Landers MB, Kreiger AE: The ora serrata in the adult human eye. Arch Ophthalmol 80:3–20, 1968

Dentate Processes and Meridional Folds

Eisner G: Zur spaltlampenmikroskopischer Ora serrata und Pars plana Corporis ciliaris. Graefes Arch Klin Exp Ophthalmol 177:232–47, 1969

Rutnin U, Schepens CL: Fundus appearance in normal eyes. II. The standard peripheral fundus and developmental variations. Am J Ophthalmol 64:840–52, 1967

Schepens CL: The standard peripheral fundus and its variations. In Retinal Detachment and Allied Diseases, vol 1. Philadelphia, Saunders, 1983, pp 134–61

Spencer LM, Foos RY, Straatsma BR: Meridional folds and meridional complexes of the peripheral retina. Trans Am Acad Ophthalmol Otolaryngol 73:204–21, 1969

Spencer LM, Foos RY, Straatsma BR: Enclosed bays of the ora serrata. Arch Ophthalmol 83:421–5, 1970

Spencer LM, Foos RY, Straatsma BR: Meridional folds, meridional complexes, and associated abnormalities of

the peripheral retina. Am J Ophthalmol 70:697–714, 1970

Straatsma BR, Landers MB, Kreiger AE: The ora serrata in the adult human eye. Arch Ophthalmol 80:3–20, 1968

Teng CC, Katzin HM: An anatomic study of the retina. Part III: Congenital retinal rosettes. Am J Ophthalmol 36:169–85, 1953

Granular Tissue (Tags) and Zonular Traction Tufts

Byer NE: Cystic retinal tufts and their relationship to retinal detachment. Arch Ophthalmol 99:1788–90, 1981

Foos RY: Zonular traction tufts of the peripheral retina in cadaver eyes. Arch Ophthalmol 82:620–32, 1969

Foos RY: Vitreoretinal juncture: Topographical variations. Invest Ophthalmol 11:801–08, 1972

Foos R: Vitreous base, retinal tufts, and retinal tears: Pathogenic relationships. In Retina Congress. Pruett RC, Regan CDJ (eds): New York, Appleton-Century-Crofts, 1974, pp 259–280

Foos RY, Allen RA: Retinal tears and lesser lesions of the peripheral retina in autopsy eyes. Am J Ophthalmol 64:643–55, 1967

Okun E: Gross and microscopic pathology in autopsy eyes. III. Retinal breaks without detachment. Am J Ophthalmol 51:369–91, 1961

Rutnin U, Schepens CL: Fundus appearance in normal eyes. II. The standard peripheral fundus and developmental variations. Am J Ophthalmol 64:840–54, 1967

Rutnin U, Schepens CL: Fundus appearance in normal eyes. IV: Retinal breaks and other findings. Am J Ophthalmol 64:1063–78, 1967

Schepens CL: The standard peripheral fundus and its variations. In Schepens CL: Retinal Detachment and Allied Diseases, vol 1. Philadelphia, Saunders, 1983, pp 134–61

Spencer LM, Straatsma BR, Foos RY: Tractional degenerations of the peripheral retina. In New Orleans Academy of Ophthalmology: Symposium of the Retina and Retinal Surgery. St. Louis, Mosby, 1969, pp 103–27

Straatsma BR, Foos RY: Part II. Peripheral retinal disorders. Classification. In L'Esperance Jr FA (ed): Current Diagnosis and Management of Chorioretinal Diseases. St. Louis, Mosby, 1977, pp 97–118

Teng CC, Katzin HM: An anatomic study

of the periphery of the retina. Part I. Nonpigmented epithelial cell proliferation and hole formation. Am J Ophthalmol 34:1237–48, 1951

Teng CC, Katzin HM: An anatomic study of the periphery of the retina. Part III: Congenital retinal rosettes. Am J Ophthalmol 36:169–85, 1953

Ora Serrata Pearls

Lonn LI, Smith TR: Ora serrata pearls. Arch Ophthalmol 77:809–13, 1967

Rutnin U, Schepens CL: Fundus appearance in normal eyes. IV: Retinal breaks and other findings. Am J Ophthalmol 64:1063–78, 1967

Samuels B: Opacities of the vitreous. Trans Ophthalmol Soc UK 50:414, 1930

Trophic Retinal Degenerations

Vitreous Base Excavations (Retinal Erosions)

Foos RY, Allen RA: Retinal tears and lesser lesions of the peripheral retina in autopsy eyes. Am J Ophthalmol 64:643–55, 1967

Foos RY, Spencer LM, Straatsma BR: Trophic degenerations of the peripheral retina. In New Orleans Academy of Ophthalmology: Symposium on Retina and Retinal Surgery. St. Louis, Mosby, 1969, pp 90–102

Rutnin U, Schepens CL: Fundus appearance in normal eyes. III: Peripheral degenerations. Am J Ophthalmol 64(6): 1040–62, 1967

Straatsma BR, Foos RY: Part II. Peripheral Retinal Disorders. Classification. In L'Esperance Jr FA (ed): Current Diagnosis and Management of Chorioretinal Diseases. St. Louis, Mosby, 1977, pp 97–118

Retinal Holes

Foos RY, Allen RA: Retinal tears and lesser lesions of the peripheral retina in autopsy eyes. Am J Ophthalmol 64:643–55, 1967

Foos RY, Spencer LM, Straatsma BR: Trophic degenerations of the peripheral retina. In New Orleans Academy of Ophthalmology: Symposium on Retina and Retinal Surgery. St. Louis, Mosby, 1969, pp 90–102

Hanssen R: Beitrag zur Histologie des myopischen Auges, insbesondere zur Luckenbildung in der Retina und zur Entstehung der Netzhautablösung.

Klin Monatsbl Augenheilkd 63:295–336, 1919

Okun E: Gross and microscopic pathology in autopsy eyes. Part III. Retinal breaks without detachment. Am J Ophthalmol 51:369–91, 1961

Rutnin V, Schepens CL: Fundus appearance in normal eyes. IV. Retinal breaks and other findings. Am J Ophthalmol 64:1063–78, 1967

Schepens CL: Retinal Detachment and Allied Diseases, vol I. Philadelphia, Saunders, 1983, pp 39, 158–60

Straatsma BR, Foos RY: Part II. Peripheral Retinal Disorders. Classification. In L'Esperance Jr FA (ed): Current Diagnosis and Management of Chorioretinal Diseases. St. Louis, Mosby, 1977, pp 97–118

Teng CC, Katzin HM: An anatomic study of the peripheral retina. II. Peripheral cystoid degeneration of the retina; Formation of cysts and holes. Am J Ophthalmol 36:29–39, 1953

Typical and Reticular Cystoid Degeneration

Foos RY, Feman SS: Reticular cystoid degeneration of the peripheral retina. Am J Ophthalmol 69:392–403, 1970

Gottinger W: Rasterelektronen mikroskopische Befunde bei peripheren cystoiden Degeneration. Dtsch Ophthalmol Ges 74:147–9, 1967

O'Malley PF, Allen RA: Peripheral cystoid degeneration of the retina. Arch Ophthalmol 77:769–76, 1967

Rutnin U, Schepens CL: Fundus appearance in normal eyes. III: Peripheral degenerations. Am J Ophthalmol 64:1040–62, 1967

Schepens CL: Retinal Detachment and Allied Diseases, vol 1. Philadelphia, Saunders, 1983, pp 141–53

Straatsma BR, Foos RY: Part II. Peripheral retinal disorders. Classification. In L'Esperance Jr FA (ed): Current Diagnosis and Management of Chorioretinal Diseases. St. Louis, Mosby, 1977, pp 97–118

Teng CC, Katzin HM: An anatomic study of the peripheral retina. II. Peripheral cystoid degeneration of the retina, formation of cysts and holes. Am J Ophthalmol 36:29–49, 1953

Acquired Typical and Reticular Degenerative Retinoschisis

Byer NE: Clinical study of senile retinoschisis. Arch Ophthalmol 79:36–44, 1986

Byer NE: The natural history of senile retinoschisis. Trans Am Acad Ophthalmol Otolaryngol 81:458–71, 1976

Foos RY: Senile retinoschisis. Relation to cystoid degeneration. Trans Am Acad Ophthalmol Otolaryngol 74:33–51, 1970

Francois J: Heredity in Ophthalmology. St. Louis, Mosby, 1961, pp 489–94

Gottinger W: Senile Retinoschisis. Stuttgart, Thieme, 1978

Hagler WS, Woldoff HS: Retinal detachment in relation to senile retinoschisis. Trans Am Acad Ophthalmol Otolaryngol 77:99–113, 1973

Hirose T, Marcil G, Schepens CL, Freeman HM: Acquired retinoschisis: Observations and treatment. In Pruett RC, Regan CDJ (eds): Retina Congress. New York, Appleton-Century-Crofts, 1972, pp 489–504

Rutnin U, Schepens CL: Fundus appearance in normal eyes. III: Peripheral degenerations. Am J Ophthalmol 64:1040–62, 1967

Schepens CL: Retinal Detachment and Allied Diseases, vol 2. Philadelphia, Saunders, 1983, pp 557–68

Shea M, Schepens CL, von Pirquet SR: I. Senile type: A clinical report of one hundred and seven cases. Arch Ophthalmol 63:1–9, 1960

Straatsma BR, Foos RY: Typical and reticular degenerative retinoschisis. Am J Ophthalmol 75:551–75, 1973

Tasman W, Shields J: Degenerative conditions. In Disorders of the Peripheral Fundus. Hagerstown, MD, Harper & Row, 1980, pp 172–6

Tolentino FI, Schepens CL, Freeman HM: Vitreoretinal Disorders: Diagnosis and Management. Philadelphia, Saunders, 1976, pp 360–5

Zimmerman LE, Spencer WH: The pathologic anatomy of retinoschisis, with a report of two cases diagnosed clinically as malignant melanoma. Arch Ophthalmol 63:10–19, 1960

Paving-Stone (Cobblestone) Degeneration

O'Malley PF, Allen RA, Straatsma BR, O'Malley CC: Paving-Stone degeneration of the retina. Arch Ophthalmol 73:169–182, 1965

Rutnin U, Schepens CL: Fundus appearance in normal eyes. III: Peripheral degenerations. Am J Ophthalmol 64: 1042–62, 1967

Schepens CL: Cobblestone degeneration of the retina. In Kimura SJ, Cagill WM

(eds): Retinal Diseases. Symposium on Differential Diagnostic Problems of Posterior Uveitis. Philadelphia, Lea & Febiger, 1966, pp 195–203

Schepens CL: Retinal Detachment and Allied Diseases, vol 1. Philadelphia, Saunders, 1983, pp 154–5

Straatsma BR, Allen RA, O'Malley P, et al: Pathologic and clinical manifestations of paving stone degeneration of the retina. In McPherson A (ed): New and Controversial Aspects of Retinal Detachment. New York, Harper & Row, 1968, pp 76–99

Straatsma BR, Foos RY: Part II. Peripheral retinal disorders. Classification. In L'Esperance Jr FA (ed): Current Diagnosis and Management of Chorioretinal Diseases. St. Louis, Mosby, 1977, pp 97–118

Peripheral Tapetochoroidal (Honeycomb) Degeneration

Foos RY, Spencer LM, Straatsma BR: Trophic degenerations of the peripheral retina. In New Orleans Academy of Ophthalmology: Symposium on Retina and Retinal Surgery. St. Louis, Mosby, 1969, pp 90–102

Rutnin U, Schepens CL: Fundus appearance in normal eyes. III: Peripheral degenerations. Am J Ophthalmol 64:1042–62, 1967

Straatsma BR, Foos RY: Part II. Peripheral Retinal Disorders. Classification. In L'Esperance Jr FA (ed): Current Diagnosis and Management of Chorioretinal Diseases. St. Louis, Mosby, 1977, pp 97–118

Equatorial Drusen

Bird A: Bruch's Membrane Degenerations. I. Disciform macular degeneration. In Archer DB (ed): Krill's Hereditary Retinal and Choroidal Diseases, vol 2: Clinical Characteristics. Hagerstown, MD, Harper & Row, 1977, pp 825–49

Farkas TG, Krial AE, Sylvester VM, et al: Familial and secondary drusen: Histologic and functional correlations. Trans Am Acad Ophthalmol Otolaryngol 75:333–43, 1971

Frakas TG, Sylvester VM, Archer D, et al: The histochemistry of drusen. Am J Ophthalmol 71:1206–15, 1971

Gass JDM: Drusen and disciform macular detachment and degeneration. Arch Ophthalmol 90:206–17, 1973

Hogan MJ: Role of the retinal pigment epithelium in macular disease. Trans

Am Acad Ophthalmol Otolaryngol 76:69–80, 1972

Krill AE, Klien BA: Flecked retina syndrome. Arch Ophthalmol 4:496–508, 1965

Lonn LI, Smith TR: Ora serrata pearls. Arch Ophthalmol 77:809–13, 1967

Tasman W, Shields JA: Disorders of the Peripheral Fundus. Hagerstown, MD, Harper & Row, 1980, pp 183–5

Tractional Retinal Degenerations

Anatomic Classification of Retinal Tears

Foos RY: Tears of the peripheral retina: Pathogenesis, incidence and classification in autopsy eyes. Mod Probl Ophthalmol 15:68–81, 1975

Foos RY: Postoral peripheral retinal tears. Ann Ophthalmol 6:679–87, 1977

Sigelman J: Vitreous base classification of retinal tears: Clinical application (review). Surv Ophthalmol 25(2): 59–74, 1980

Partial-Thickness Peripheral Retinal Tears

Foos RY, Allen RA: Retinal tears and lesser lesions of the peripheral retina in autopsy eyes. Am J Ophthalmol 64:643–55, 1967

Gärtner J: Histologische Beobachtungen über physiologische vitreovasculäre Adhärenzen. Klin Monatsbl Augenheilkd 141:530, 1962

Gärtner J: Über persistierende netzhautadhärente glaskörperstränge und vitreoretinale Gefässanastomosen. Graefes Arch Ophthalmol 167:103, 1964

Rieger H: Zur Histologie der Glaskörperabhebung. II. Über die Beziehungen des abgehobenen Glaskörpers zur Netzhaut. Graefe's Arch Ophthalmol 146(4): 447–62, 1943

Rutnin U, Schepens CL: Fundus appearance in normal eyes. IV. Retinal breaks and other findings. Am J Ophthalmol 64: 1063–78, 1967

Spencer LM, Foos RY: Paravascular vitreoretinal attachments: Role in retinal tears. Arch Ophthalmol 84:557–64, 1970

Spencer LM, Straatsma BR, Foos RY: Tractional degenerations of the peripheral retina. In New Orleans Academy of Ophthalmology: Symposium of the Retina and Retinal Surgery. St. Louis, Mosby, 1969, pp 103–27

Straatsma BR, Foos RY: Part II. Peripheral retinal disorders. Classification. In L'Es-

perance Jr FA (ed): Current Diagnosis and Management of Chorioretinal Diseases. St. Louis, Mosby, 1977, pp 97–118

Full-Thickness Peripheral Retinal Tears

Arentsen JJ, Welch RB: Retinal detachment in the young individual: A survey of 100 cases seen at the Wilmer Institute. J Pediatr Ophthalmol 11:198–202, 1974

Ashrafzadeh MT, Schepens CL, Elzeneiny IT: Aphakic and phakic retinal detachment. Arch Ophthalmol 89:476–83, 1973

Benson WE, Grand MG, Okun E: Aphakic retinal detachment. Arch Ophthalmol 93:245–9, 1975

Byer NE: Clinical study of retinal breaks. Trans Am Acad Ophthalmol Otolaryngol 71:461–73, 1967

Colyear BM, Pischel DK: Clinical tears without detachment. Am J Ophthalmol 41:773–92, 1956

Cox MS, Schepens CL, Freeman HM: Retinal detachment due to ocular contusion. Arch Ophthalmol 76:678–85, 1966

Davis MD: The natural history of retinal breaks. Arch Ophthalmol 92:183–94, 1974

Delori F, Pomerantzeff O, Cox MS: Deformation of the globe under high-speed impact: Its relation to contusion injuries. Invest Ophthalmol 8:290–301, 1969

Everett WG, Katzin D: Meridional distribution of retinal breaks in aphakic retinal detachment. Am J Ophthalmol 66:928–32, 1968

Foos RY: Zonular traction tufts of the peripheral retina in cadaver eyes. Arch Ophthalmol 82:620–32, 1969

Foos RY: Posterior vitreous detachment. Trans Am Acad Ophthalmol Otolaryngol 76:480–97, 1972

Foos RY: Vitreous base, retinal tufts and retinal tears: Pathogenetic relationships. In Pruett RC, Regan CDJ (eds): Retina Congress. New York, Appleton-Century-Crofts, 1972, pp 259–80

Foos RY: Tears of the peripheral retina: Pathogenesis, incidence and classification in autopsy eyes. Mod Probl Ophthalmol 15:68–81, 1975

Foos RY: Postoral peripheral retinal tears. Ann Ophthalmol 6:679–87, 1977

Hauer Y, Barkay S: Vitreous detachment in aphakic eyes. Br J Ophthalmol 48:341–3, 1964

Heller MD, Straatsma BR, Foos RY: Detachment of the posterior vitreous in phakic and aphakic eyes. Secondary de-

tachment of the retina. Mod Probl Ophthalmol 10:23–36, 1972

Jaffe NA: Complications of acute posterior vitreous detachment. Arch Ophthalmol 79:568–71, 1968

Norton EWD: Retinal detachment in aphakia. Trans Am Ophthalmol Soc 61:770–89, 1963

Robertson DM, Curtin VT, Norton EWD: Avulsed retinal vessels with retinal breaks. Arch Ophthalmol 85:669–72, 1971

Rutnin U, Schepens CL: Fundus appearance in normal eyes. IV: Retinal breaks and other findings. Am J Ophthalmol 64:1063–78, 1967

Scheie HG, Morse PH, Aminlari A: Incidence of retinal detachment following cataract extraction. Arch Ophthalmol 89:293–5, 1973

Schepens CL: Pathogenesis of traumatic rhegmatogenous retinal detachment In Freeman HM (ed): Ocular Trauma. New York, Appleton-Century-Crofts, 1979, pp 273–84

Tasman W: Posterior vitreous detachment and peripheral retinal breaks. Trans Am Acad Ophthalmol Otolaryngol 72:217–24, 1968

Tasman W: Peripheral retinal changes following blunt trauma. Trans Am Ophthalmol Soc 70:190–8, 1972

Tasman W, Shields JA: Disorders of the peripheral fundus. Hagerstown, MD, Harper & Row, 1980, pp 205–6

Weidenthal DT, Schepens CL: Peripheral fundus changes associated with ocular contusion. Am J Ophthalmol 62:465–77, 1966

Retinal Dialyses (Juvenile)

Arentsen JJ, Welch RB: Retinal detachment in the young individual: A survey of 100 cases seen at the Wilmer Institute. J Pediatr Ophthalmol 11:198–202, 1974

Benson WE, Nantawan P, Morse PH: Characteristics and prognosis of retinal detachments with demarcation lines. Am J Ophthalmol 84:641–4, 1977

Black RK, Davies EWG: The management of retinal dialysis. Trans Ophthalmol Soc UK 87:317–33, 1967

Chignell AH: Retinal dialysis. Br J Ophthalmol 57:572–7, 1972

Cox MS: Retinal breaks caused by nonperforation trauma at the point of impact. Trans Am Ophthalmol Soc 78:413–66, 1980

Cox MS, Schepens CL, Freeman HM: Retinal detachment due to ocular contu-sion. Arch Ophthalmol 76:678–85, 1966

Duke-Elder S, Dobree JH: System of Ophthalmology, vol 10: Diseases of the Retina. London, Henry Kimpton, 1967, pp 789–90

Freeman HM, Cox MS, Schepens CL: Traumatic retinal detachments. Int Ophthalmol Clin 14(4):151–70, 1974

Hagler WS, North AW: Retinal dialyses and retinal detachment. Arch Ophthalmol 79:376–88, 1968

Hilton GF, Norton EWD: Juvenile retinal detachment. Mod Probl Ophthalmol 8:325–41, 1969

Hudson JR: Retinal detachment in children. Trans Ophthalmol Soc UK 85:79–91, 1965

Schepens CL: Pathogenesis of traumatic rhegmatogenous retinal detachment. In Freeman HM (ed): Ocular Trauma. New York, Appleton-Century-Crofts, 1979, pp 273–84

Tasman W: Peripheral retinal changes following blunt trauma. Trans Am Ophthalmol Soc 70:190–8, 1972

Tasman W: Retinal dialysis following blunt trauma. In Freeman HM (ed): Ocular Trauma. New York, Appleton-Century-Crofts, 1979, pp 295–9

Verdaguer TJ, Rojas B, Lechuga M: Genetical studies in nontraumatic retinal dialysis. Mod Probl Ophthalmol 15:34–9, 1975

Watzke RC: The ophthalmoscopic sign "white-with-pressure." Arch Ophthalmol 66:812–23, 1961

Weidenthal DT, Schepens CL: Peripheral fundus changes associated with ocular contusion. Am J Ophthalmol 62:465–77, 1966

Winslow R, Tasman W: Juvenile retinal detachment. Trans Am Acad Ophthalmol Otolaryngol 85:607–18, 1978

Giant Retinal Tears

Freeman HM: Current management of giant retinal breaks. In New Orleans Academy of Ophthalmology: Symposium on Retina and Retinal Surgery. St. Louis, Mosby, 1969, pp 171–83

Freeman HM: Current management of giant retinal breaks. In Pruett RC, Regan CDJ (eds): Retina Congress. New York, Appleton-Century-Crofts, 1972, pp 435–63

Freeman HM: Vitreous surgery. X. Current status of vitreous surgery in cases of rhegmatogenous retinal detachment. Trans Am Acad Ophthalmol Otolaryngol 77:202–15, 1973

Freeman HM: Fellow eyes of giant retinal breaks. Trans Am Ophthalmol Soc 76:343–82, 1978

Glasspool MG, Kanski JJ: Prophylaxis in giant tears. Trans Ophthalmol Soc UK 93:363–71, 1973

Hovland KR, Schepens CL, Freeman HM: Developmental giant tears associated with lens coloboma. Arch Ophthalmol 80:325–31, 1968

Kanski J: Giant retinal tears. Am J Ophthalmol 78:846–52, 1975

Lincoff HA, Kreissig I, La Franco F: Large retinal tears. Am J Ophthalmol 84:501–08, 1977

Machemer R, Allen AW: Retinal tears 180 degrees and greater. Management with vitrectomy and intravitreal gas. Arch Ophthalmol 94:1340–6, 1976

Norton EWD: Intra-ocular gas in the management of selected retinal detachments. Trans Am Acad Ophthalmol Otolaryngol 77:85–98, 1973

Norton EWD, Aaberg TM, Fung W, et al: Giant retinal tears. Am J Ophthalmol 68:1011–21, 1969

Schepens CL, Freeman HM: Current management of giant retinal breaks. Trans Am Acad Ophthalmol Otolaryngol 71:474–87, 1967

Scott JD: Equatorial giant tears affected by massive vitreous retraction. Trans Ophthalmol Soc UK 96:309–12, 1976

Scott JD: A rationale for the use of liquid silicone. Trans Ophthalmol Soc UK 97:235–7, 1977

Trophic and Tractional Retinal Degenerations

White-with- or -without-Pressure

Goldbaum MH, Joondeph N, Huamonte FU, et al: White-with-pressure or white-without-pressure lesions. In Peyman GA, Sanders DR, Goldberg MF (eds): Principles and Practice of Ophthalmology. Philadelphia, Saunders, 1980, pp 1027–8

Grignolo A: Ophthalmoscopy and other methods of examination. In Schepens CL, Regan CDJ (eds): Controversial Aspects of the Management of Retinal Detachment. Boston, Little, Brown, 1965, pp 2–28

Karlin DB, Curtin BJ: Axial length measurements and peripheral fundus changes in the myopic eye. In Pruett RC, Regan CDJ (eds): Retinal Congress. New York, Appleton-Century-Crofts, 1972, pp 629–42

Nagpal KC, Huamonte FU, Constantaras A, et al: Migratory white without pressure retinal lesions. Arch Ophthalmol 94:576–9, 1976

Rutnin U, Schepens CL: Fundus appearance in normal eyes. IV. Retinal breaks and other findings. Am J Ophthalmol 64:1063–78, 1967

Schepens CL: Subclinical retinal detachments. Arch Ophthalmol 47:593–608, 1952

Watzke RC: The ophthalmic sign white-with-pressure. A clinicopathologic correlation. Arch Ophthalmol 66:812–23, 1961

Snail-Track Retinal Degeneration

Aaberg TM, Stevens TR: Snail track degeneration of the retina. Am J Ophthalmol 73:370–6, 1972

Byer NE: Clinical study of lattice degeneration of the retina. Trans Am Acad Ophthalmol Otolaryngol 69:1064–77, 1965

Cibis PA: Vitre et décollement de rétine. Arch Ophtalmol 25:627–37, 1965

Deutman A: Vitreoretinal dystrophies. In Archer DB (ed): Krill's Hereditary Retinal and Choroidal Diseases, vol 2: Clinical Characteristics.

Gonin J: Le pathogénie du décollement spontané de la rétine. Ann Oculist 132:30, 1904

Gonin J: Le Décollement de la Rétine, Pathogénie-Traitment. Lausanne, Librairie Payot, 1934

Lattice Retinal Degeneration

Allen RA, Straatsma BR: The pathology of lattice degeneration of the retina. Mod Probl Ophthalmol 4:49–66, 1966

Byer NE: Prognosis of asymptomatic retinal breaks. Arch Ophthalmol 92:208–10, 1974

Byer NE: Changes in and prognosis of lattice degeneration of the retina, Trans Am Acad Ophthalmol Otolaryngol 78:114–25, 1974

Byer NE: A clinical definition of lattice degeneration of the retina and its variations. Mod Probl Ophthalmol 15:58–67, 1975

Byer NE: Lattice degeneration of the retina (a review). Surv Ophthalmol 23:213–48, 1979

Bonuk M, Butler FC: An autopsy study of lattice degeneration, retinal breaks and retinal pits. In McPherson A (ed): New and Controversial Aspects of Retinal

Detachment. New York, Harper & Row, 1968, pp 59–75

Davis MD: Natural history of retinal breaks without detachment. Arch Ophthalmol 92:183–94, 1974

Deutman AF: Vitreoretinal dystrophies. In Archer DB (ed): Krill's Hereditary Retinal and Choroidal Diseases, vol 2: Clinical Characteristics. Hagerstown, MD, Harper & Row, 1977, pp 1093–6

Dumas J, Schepens CL: Chorioretinal lesions predisposing to retinal breaks. Am J Ophthalmol 61:620–30, 1966

Gonin J: Le Décollement de la Rétine, Pathogénie Traitement. Lausanne, Librairie Payot, 1934

Okun E: Gross and microscopic pathology in autopsy eyes. Part III. Retinal breaks without detachment. Am J Ophthalmol 51:369–91, 1961

Rutnin U, Schepens CL: Fundus appearance of normal eyes. III: Peripheral degenerations. Am J Ophthalmol 64(6):1040–62, 1967

Schepens CL: Symposium Retinal Detachment: Diagnostic and prognostic factors as found in preoperative examination. Trans Am Acad Ophthalmol Otolaryngol 56:398–418, 1952

Straatsma BR, Allen RA: Lattice degeneration of the retina. Trans Am Acad Ophthalmol Otolaryngol 66:600–12, 1962

Straatsma BR, Zeegen PD, Foos RY, et al: 30th Edward Jackson Memorial Lecture: Lattice degeneration of the retina. Trans Am Acad Ophthalmol Otolaryngol 78:87–113, 1974

Straatsma BR, Zeegen PD, Foos RY, et al: Lattice degeneration of the retina. Am J Ophthalmol 77:619–49, 1974

Streeten BW, Bert M: Retinal surface in lattice degeneration of the retina. Am J Ophthalmol 74:1201–09, 1972

Tillery WV, Lucier AC: Round atrophic holes in lattice degeneration – An important cause of phakic retinal detachment. Trans Am Ophthalmol, Otolaryngol 81:509–18, 1976

Hereditary Vitreoretinal Degenerations

Wagner's Hereditary Vitreoretinal Degeneration and Stickler's Syndrome

Alexander RL, Shea M: Wagner's disease. Arch Ophthalmol 74:310–18, 1965

Blair NP, Albert DM, Liberfarb RM, Hirose T: Hereditary progressive arthro-ophthalmopathy of Stickler. Am J Ophthalmol 88:876–88, 1979

Böhringer HR, Dieterle P, Landolt E: Zur Klinik und Pathologie der Degeneratio hyaloideo-retinalis hereditaria (Wagner). Ophthalmologica 139:330–8, 1960

Hagler WS, Crosswell HH Jr: Radial paravascular chorioretinal degeneration and retinal detachment. Trans Am Acad Ophthalmol Otolaryngol 72:203–16, 1968

Hirose T, Lee KY, Schepens CL: Wagner's hereditary vitreo-retinal degeneration and retinal detachment. Arch Ophthalmol 89:176–85, 1973

Hirose T, Miyake Y: Pigmentary paravenous chorioretinal degeneration: Fundus appearance and retinal functions. Annals of Ophthalmology 11:(5), 709–718, 1979

Jansen L: Degeneratio hyaloideo-retinalis hereditaria. Ophthalmologica 144:458–64, 1962

Knobloch WH: Inherited hyaloideo-retinopathy and skeletal dysplasia. Trans Am Ophthalmol Soc 73:417–51, 1976

Knobloch WH, Layer JM: Clefting syndromes associated with retinal detachment. Am J Ophthalmol 73:517–30, 1972

Liberfarb RM, Hirose T, Holmes LB: The Wagner-Stickler syndrome: A genetic study of twenty-two families. J Pediatr 99:394–9, 1981

Schepens CL: Retinal Detachment and Allied Diseases, vol 2. Philadelphia, Saunders, 1983, pp 599–614

Schreiner RL, McAlister WH, Marshall RE, Shearer WT: Stickler syndrome in a pedigree of Pierre Robin syndrome. Am J Dis Child 126:86–90, 1973

Stickler GB, Belau PG, Farrell FJ, et al: Hereditary progressive arthro-ophthalmopathy. Mayo Clin Proc 40:433–55, 1965

Stickler GB, Pugh DG: Hereditary progressive arthro-ophthalmopathy. II. Additional observations on vertebral abnormalities, a hearing defect and a report of a similar case. Mayo Clin Proc 42:495–500, 1967

Wagner H: Ein bisher unbekanntes Erbleiden des Auges (Degeneratio hyaloideo-retinalis hereditaria) beobachtet im Kanton Zurich. Klin Monatsbl Augenheilkd 100:840–57, 1938

Juvenile Retinoschisis

Burns RP, Lovrien FW, Cibis AB: Juvenile sex-linked retinoschisis: Clinical and genetic studies. Trans Am Acad Ophthalmol Otolaryngol 75:1011–21, 1971

Brodrick JD, Wyatt HT: Hereditary sex-linked retinoschisis. Br J Ophthalmol 57:551–9, 1973

Ede CH, Wilson RJ: Juvenile retinoschisis. Br J Ophthalmol 57:560–2, 1973

Kraushar MF, Schepens CL, Kaplan JA, Freeman HM: Congenital retinoschisis. In Bellows JG (ed): Contemporary Ophthalmology Honoring Sir Stewart Duke-Elder. Baltimore, Williams & Wilkins, 1972, pp 265–90

Lewis RA, Lee GB, Martonyi CL, et al: Familial foveal retinoschisis. Arch Ophthalmol 95:1190–6, 1977

Manschot WA: Pathology of hereditary juvenile retinoschisis. Arch Ophthalmol 88:131–8, 1972

Sabates FN: Juvenile retinoschisis. Am J Ophthalmol 62:683–8, 1966

Sarin LK, Green WR, Daile EG: Juvenile retinoschisis. Congenital vascular veils and hereditary retinoschisis. Am J Ophthalmol 57:793–6, 1964

Schepens CL: Retinal Detachment and Allied Diseases, vol 2. Philadelphia, Saunders, 1983, pp 568–88

Tasman W, Shields JA: Disorders of the Peripheral Fundus. Hagerstown, MD, Harper & Row, 1980, pp 36–41

Tolentino FI, Schepens CL, Freeman HM: Vitreoretinal Disorders: Diagnosis and Management. Philadelphia, Saunders, 1976, pp 249–59

Yanoff M, Rahn EK, Zimmerman LE: Histopathology of juvenile retinoschisis. Arch Ophthalmol 79:49–53, 1968

Zimmerman LE, Naumann G: The pathology of retinoschisis. In McPherson A (ed): New and Controversial Aspects of Retinal Detachment. New York, Hoeber / Harper & Row, 1968, pp 400–23

Goldman-Favre Disease

Blanck MF, Polliot L, Bernard P: La dégénérescence hyaloide tapéto-rétinienne de Goldmann et Favré à propos d'un cas. Bull Mem Soc Fr Ophtal 86:242–5, 1973

Carr RE, Siegel JM: The vitreo-tapeto-retinal degenerations. Arch Ophthalmol 84:436–45, 1970

Deutman AF: Vitreoretinal dystrophies. In Archer DB (ed): Krill's Hereditary Retinal and Choroidal Diseases, vol 2: Clinical Characteristics. Hagerstown, MD, Harper & Row, 1977, pp 1062–8

Favre M, Goldmann H: Zur Genese der hinteren Glaskörperabhebung. Ophthalmologica 132:87–97, 1957

Favre M: A propos de deux cas de dégénérescence hyaloidéo-rétinienne. Ophthalmologica. 135:604–09, 1958

Feiler-Ofry V, Adams A, Regenbogen L: Hereditary vitreoretinal degeneration and night blindness. Am J Ophthalmol 67:553–8, 1969

Francois J, de Rouck A, Cambie E: Dégénérescence hyaloidéo-tapéto-rétinienne de Goldmann-Favre. Ophthalmologica 168:81–96, 1974

Gerhard JP, Bronner A, Flament J: Rétinopathie pigmentaire et décollement de la rétine. Bull Soc Ophtalmol Fr 72:133–6, 1972

Goldmann H: Biomicroscopic du corps vitré et du fond d'œil. Rapp Soc Fr Ophtalmol, pp 164–9, 1957

Ricci A: Clinique et transmission héréditaire des dégénérescences vitréo-rétiniennes. Bull Soc Ophtalmol Fr 61:618–62, 1961

Stankovic I, Kecmanovic Z, Drincic V: Contribution à la connaissance de l'hérédité de la dégénérescence hyaloidéo-tapéto-rétinienne de Favre-Goldmann. Bull Mem Soc Fr Ophtalmol 86:246–50, 1973

Familial Exudative Vitreoretinopathy

Criswick VG, Schepens CL: Familial exudative vitreoretinopathy. Am J Ophthalmol 68:578–94, 1969

Deutman AF: Vitreoretinal dystrophies. In Archer DB (ed): Krill's Hereditary Retinal and Choroidal Diseases, vol 2: Clinical Characteristics. Hagerstown, MD, Harper & Row, 1977, pp 1084–92

Gow J, Oliver GL: Familial exudative vitreoretinopathy. An expanded view. Am J Ophthalmol 86:150–5, 1971

Snowflake Degeneration

Deutman AF: Vitreoretinal dystrophies. In Archer DB (ed): Krill's Hereditary Retinal and Choroidal Diseases. Hagerstown, MD, Harper & Row, 1977, pp 1097–1100

Hirose T, Lee KY, Schepens CL: Snowflake degeneration in hereditary vitreoretinal degeneration. Am J Ophthalmol 77:143–53, 1974

Hirose T, Wolf E, Schepens CL: Retinal functions in snowflake degeneration. Ann Ophthalmol 12:1135–46, 1980

Schepens CL: Retinal Detachment and Allied Diseases, vol 2. Philadelphia, Saunders, 1983, pp 614–15

Systemic Conditions Associated with Vitreoretinal Degeneration

Marfan's Syndrome

Archard C: Arachnodactylie. Bull Mem Soc Med Hop Paris 19:834–40, 1902

Franceschetti A, Francois J, Babel J: Les Hérédodégénérescences Choriorétiniennes (Dégénérescences Tapeto-Rétiniennes), vol 1, 2. Paris, Masson, 1963

Heilmann K, Suschke J, Murken JD: Marfan-Syndrome. Ophthalmologische, klinische, biochemische und genetische Untersuchungen. Ber. 70. Bericht über die Zusammenkunft der Deutschen Ophthalmologischen Gesellschaft, Heidelberg, 1969. München, Bergmann, 1970, pp 457, 599

Lloyd RI: The clinical course of the eye complications of arachrodactylia. Trans Am Ophthalmol Soc 45:342, 1947

Marfan B: Un cas de déformation congénitale des quatre membres, plus prononcée aux extrémités, caractérisée par l'allongement des os avec un certain degré d'amincissement. Bull Med Soc Hop Paris 13:220–6, 1896

Schepens CL: Retinal Detachment and Allied Diseases, vol 1. Philadelphia, Saunders, 1983, pp 268–70

Sinclair RJG, Kitchin AW, Turner RWD: The Marfan Syndrome. Q J Med 29:19–46, 1960

Homocystinuria

Allen RA, Straatsma BR, Apt L, Hall MO: Ocular manifestations of Marfan's syndrome. Trans Am Acad Ophthalmol Otolaryngol 71:18–38, 1967

Carson NAJ, Dent CE, Field CMB, Gaull CE: Homocystinuria: Clinical and pathological review of ten cases. J Pediat 6:565–83, 1965

Cross HE, Jensen AD: Ocular manifestations in Marfan's syndrome and homocystinuria. Am J Ophthalmol 75:405–20, 1973

Field CMB, Carson NAJ, Cosworth DC, et al: Homocystinuria: A new disorder of metabolism. 10th International Congress of Pediatrics, Lisbon, 1962, p 274

Francois J, Gaudier B, Pruvot J: La rétine dans l'homocystinurie. Bull Soc Ophtalmol Fr 68:582–4, 1968

Francois J: Ocular manifestations in amino-acidopathies. Adv Ophthalmol 25:28, 1972

Henkind P, Ashton N: Ocular pathology in homocystinuria. Trans Ophthalmol Soc UK 85:21–38, 1965

Hudson JR: Marfan's syndrome with retinal detachment. Br J Ophthalmol 35:244–5, 1951

Lieberman TN, Podos SM, Hartstein J: Acute glaucoma, ectopia lentis, and homocystinuria. Am J Ophthalmol 61:252–5, 1966

Schmike RN, McKusick VA, Huang T, Pollack AD: Homocystinuria studies of twenty families with thirty-eight affected members. JAMA 193:711–19, 1965

Spaeth GL, Barber GW: Homocystinuria, its ocular manifestation. J Pediat Ophthalmol 3:42–8, 1966

Ehlers-Danlos Syndrome

Beighton P: X-linked inheritance in the Ehlers-Danlos syndrome. Br Med J 2:409–11, 1968

Beighton P: Serious ophthalmological complications in the Ehlers-Danlos syndrome. Br J Ophthalmol 54:263–8, 1970

Bossu A, Lambrechts J: Manifestations oculaires du syndrome d'Ehlers-Danlos. Ann Oculist (Paris) 187:227–36, 1954

Cottini GB: Concurrence of the Groenblad-Strandberg syndrome and the Ehlers-Danlos syndrome. Acta Derm 29:544–9, 1949

Danlos H: Un cas de cutis laxa avec tumeurs par contusion chromique des coudes et des genoux. Bull Soc Fr Derm Syphilo 19:70, 1908

Durham DG: Cutis hyperelastica (Ehlers-Danlos syndrome) with blue scleras, microcornea, and glaucoma. Arch Ophthalmol 49:220–1, 1953

Ehlers E: Cutis laxa. Neigung zu Hamorrhagien in der Haut, Lockerung mehrerer Artikulationen. Dermatol Wochenschr 8:173, 1899

Green WR: Angioid streaks in Ehlers-Danlos syndrome. Arch Ophthalmol 76:197, 1966

Jansen LH: The structure of the connective tissue, an explanation of the symptoms and Ehlers-Danlos syndrome. Dermatologica 110:108–20, 1955

Johnson SAM, Falls HF: Ehlers-Danlos syndrome: A clinical and genetic study. Arch Dermatol Syphilol 60:80–105, 1949

Méténier P: A propos d'un familial de maladie d'Ehlers-Danlos. Thesis. University of Algiers, 1939, p 55

Pemberton JW, Freeman HM, Schepens CL: Familial retinal detachment and the Ehlers-Danlos syndrome. Arch Ophthalmol 76:817–24, 1966

Summer GK: The Ehlers-Danlos syndrome: A review of the literature and report of a case with subgaleal hematoma and Bell's palsy. Am J Dis Child 91:419–28, 1956

Wiedermann HR: Einiges zum Syndrom von Ehlers and Danlos. Z Kinderheilkd 100:252–6, 1952

Degenerative Conditions of the Vitreous Body

Asteroid Hyalosis

Agarwal IP, Mohan M, Khosla PK, Gupta AK: Synchysis scintillians or asteroid bodies. Orient Arch Ophthalmol 1:167–70, 1963

Bard LA: Asteroid hyalitis: Relationship to diabetes and hypercholesterolemia. Am J Ophthalmol 58:239–42, 1964

Benson AH: A case of "monocular asteroid hyalitis." Trans Ophthalmol Soc UK 14:101–04, 1894

Cibis P: Vitreoretinal Pathology and Surgery in Retinal Detachment. St. Louis, Mosby, 1965, p 193

Duke-Elder WS: System of Ophthalmology, vol 11. Diseases of the Lens and the Vitreous; Glaucoma and Hypotony. London, Henry Kimpton, 1969, pp 323–8

Hatfield RE, Gastineau CF, Rucker CW: Asteroid bodies in the vitreous: Relationship to diabetes and hypercholesterolemia. Proc Mayo Clin 37:513–14, 1962

Hogan M, Zimmerman L: Ophthalmic Pathology. An Atlas and Textbook, 2nd ed. Philadelphia, Saunders, 1962, pp 62, 651

Luxemberg M, Sime D: Relationship of asteroid hyalosis to diabetes mellitus and plasma lipid levels. Am J Ophthalmol 67:406–13, 1969

March W, Shock D, O'Grady R: Composition of asteroid bodies. Invest Ophthalmol 13:701–05, 1974

Pau H: Ätiologische Betrachtungen zur Scintallatio Nivea. Ophthalmologica (Basel) 150:167–74, 1965

Rodman HI, Johnson FB, Zimmerman LE: New histopathological and histochemical observations concerning asteroid hyalitis. Arch Ophthalmol 66:552–63, 1961

Rutherford CW: Asteroid bodies in the vitreous. Arch Ophthalmol 9:106–17, 1933

Smith JL: Asteroid hyalitis: Incidence of diabetes mellitus and hypercholesterolemia. JAMA 168:891–3, 1958

VerHoeff FH: Microscopic findings in a case of asteroid hyalitis. Am J Ophthalmol 4:155–60, 1921

Synchysis Scintillans

Forsius H: Cholesterol crystals in the anterior chamber. Acta Ophthalmol 39:284–301, 1961

Hughes WL, in discussion, Bonaccalto G: Synchysis scintillans in the anterior chamber. Arch Ophthalmol 18:477, 1937

Jaffe NS: The Vitreous in Clinical Ophthalmology. St. Louis, Mosby, 1969, pp 223–6

Koby FE: Biomicroscopie du Corps Vitré. Paris, Masson, 1932, p 100

Manschot WA: Synchysis scintillans. Acta Ophthalmol 20:80–90, 1942

Michiels J, Garin P: Synchisis étincelant de la chambre antérieure. Bull Soc Belg Ophtalmol 151:455–63, 1969

Valenin F: Über die fettähnlichen Substanzen im Glasskörper des Pferdeauges. Z Physiol Chem 105:33–57, 1919

Wand M, Gorn RA: Cholesterolosis of the anterior chamber. Am J Ophthal 78:143–4, 1974

Primary Hereditary Familial Amyloidosis

Andersson R, Kassman T: Vitreous opacities in primary familial amyloidosis. Acta Ophthalmol 46:441–7, 1968

Cohen AS: Amyloidosis. N Engl J Med 277:(10)522–630; (11)574–583; (12)628–638, 1967

Crawford JB: Cotton wool exudates in systemic amyloidosis. Arch Ophthalmol 78:214–16, 1967

Cupper C: Augenbefunde bei Paramyloid. Ber Dtsch Ophthalmol Ges 56:337–9, 1951

Falls HF, Jackson J, Carey J, et al: Ocular manifestations of hereditary primary systemic amyloidosis. Arch Ophthalmol 54:660–4, 1958

Ferry AP, Lieberman TW: Bilateral amyloidosis of the vitreous body. Report of a case without systemic or familial involvement. Arch Ophthalmol 94:982–91, 1976

Franceschetti AT, Rubinowicz T: Les lésions oculaires dans l'amyloidose primaire familiale. J Genet Hum 17: 349–66, 1969

Kantarjian AD, DeJong R: Familial primary amyloidosis with nervous system involvement. Neurology 3:399–409, 1953

Kaufman HE: Primary familial

amyloidosis. Arch Ophthalmol 60:1036–43, 1959

Kaufman HE, Thomas LB: Vitreous opacities diagnostic of familial primary amyloidosis. N Engl J Med 261:1267–71, 1959

Missmahl HP, Siebner H: Chromosomen-untersuchung bei familiarer perikollagener Amyloidose. Dtsch Med Wochenschr 90:1002–4, 1965

Paton D, Duke JR: Primary familial amyloidosis. Am J Ophthalmol 61:736–47, 1966

Rukavina JG, Block WD, Jackson C, et al: Primary systemic amyloidosis: A review and an experimental, genetic, and clinical study of twenty-nine cases with particular emphasis on familial form. Medicine 35:239–334, 1956

Wong VG, McFarlin DE: Primary familial amyloidosis. Arch Ophthalmol 78:208–13, 1967

Proliferative Retinopathies

Diabetic Retinopathy

Aaberg TM: Clinical results in vitrectomy for diabetic traction retinal detachment. Am J Ophthalmol 88:246–53, 1979

Aiello LM, Beetham WP, Balodimos MC, et al: Ruby laser photocoagulation in treatment of diabetes proliferating retinopathy: Primary report. In Goldberg M, Fine S (eds): Symposium on the Treatment of Diabetic Retinopathy. Washington, DC, US Department of Health, Education, and Welfare, Public Health Service Publication No. 1890, US Government Printing Office, 1969, pp 437–63.

Benson WE, Spalter HF: Vitreous hemorrhage. A review of experimental and clinical investigations. Surv Ophthalmol 15:297–311, 1971

Benson WE, Tasman W, Duane TD: Diabetic retinopathy. In Duane TD (ed): Clinical Ophthalmology, vol III. Hagerstown, MD, Harper & Row, 1976, pp 1–24

Blankenship G: Pars plana vitrectomy for diabetic retinopathy. A report of eight years experience. Mod Probl Ophthalmol 20:376–86, 1979

Blankenship GW, Skyler JS: Diabetic retinopathy. A general survey. Diabetes Care 1:127–31, 1978

Bresnick GH, Davis MD, Myers FL, et al: Clinical pathologic correlations in diabetic retinopathy. II. Clinical and histologic appearances of retinal capillary microaneurysms. Arch Ophthal 95:1215–1220, 1977

Brotherman DP: Diabetic retinopathy. A perspective. Surv Ophthalmol 16:359–70, 1972

Burditt AF, Caird FL, Draper GJ: The natural history of diabetic retinopathy. Q J Med 37:303–17, 1968

Caird FI, Pirie A, Ramsell TG: Diabetes and the Eye. Oxford and Edinburgh, Blackwell Scientific Publications, 1968, pp 1–7

Cogan DG, Toussaint D, Kuwabara T: Retinal vascular patterns. IV. Diabetic retinopathy. Arch Ophthalmol 66:366–78, 1961

Cogan DG, Kuwabara T: Ocular microangiopathy in diabetes. In Kimura JS, Caygill WM (eds): Vascular Complications of Diabetes Mellitus. St. Louis, Mosby, 1967, pp 53–73

Davis MD: Vitreous contraction in proliferative diabetic retinopathy. Arch Ophthalmol 74:741–51, 1965

The Diabetic Retinopathy Study Research Group: Preliminary report on effects of photocoagulation therapy. Am J Ophthalmol 81:383–6, 1976

The Diabetic Retinopathy Study Research Group: Photocoagulation treatment of diabetic retinopathy: The second report of diabetic retinopathy study findings. Ophthalmology 85:82–105, 1978

The Diabetic Retinopathy Study Research Group: Four risk factors for severe visual loss in diabetic retinopathy: The third report from the diabetic retinopathy study. Arch Ophthalmol 97:654–5, 1979

The Diabetic Retinopathy Study Research Group: Protocoagulation of proliferative diabetic retinopathy: Clinical application of diabetic retinopathy study (DRS) findings. Ophthalmology 88:583–600, 1981

Dobree JH: Proliferative diabetic retinopathy. Evolution of the retinal lesions. Br J Ophthalmol 48:637–49, 1964

Irvine AR, Norton EWD: Photocoagulation for diabetic retinopathy. Am J Ophthalmol 71:437–45, 1971

Kahn HA, Bradely RF: Prevalence of diabetic retinopathy. Br J Ophthalmol 59:345–49, 1979

Keen H: The prevalence of blindness in diabetes. J R Coll Physicians London 7:53–61, 1972

Knowler WC, Bennett PH, Ballintine EJ: Increased incidence of retinopathy in diabetics with elevated blood pressure. N Engl J Med 302:645–50, 1980

Kohner EM: The evolution and natural history of diabetic retinopathy. Int Ophthalmol Clin 18:1–16, 1978

L'Esperance Jr FA, James Jr WA: Diabetic Retinopathy. Clinicial Evaluation and Management. St. Louis, Mosby, 1981, pp 89–114

Little HL: Pathogenesis. In L'Esperance FA Jr, James WA Jr (eds): Diabetic Retinopathy. Clinical Evaluation and Management. St. Louis, Mosby, 1981, pp 58–88

Mandelcorn MS, Blankenship G, Machemer R: Pars plana vitrectomy for the management of severe diabetic retinopathy. Am J Ophthalmol 81:561–70, 1976

McMeel JW: Diabetic retinopathy: Fibrotic proliferation and retinal detachment. Trans Am Ophthalmol Soc 69:440–93, 1971

Michels RG: Vitrectomy for complications of diabetic retinopathy. Arch Ophthalmol 96:237–46, 1978

Morse PH, Aminlari A, Scheie HG: Spontaneous vitreous hemorrhage. Arch Ophthalmol 92:297–8, 1974

Patz A, Schatz H, Berkow JW, et al: Macular edema – an overlooked complication of diabetic retinopathy. Trans Am Acad Ophthalmol Otolaryngol 77:34–42, 1973

Schatz H, Patz A: Cystoid maculopathy in diabetics. Arch Ophthalmol 94:761–8, 1976

Sigelman J: Diabetic maculopathy. In L'Esperance FA Jr, James WA Jr (eds): Diabetic Retinopathy. Clinical Evaluation and Management. St. Louis, Mosby, 1981, pp 191–201

Spalter HF: Photocoagulation of diabetic retinopathy. (A rationale). In Goldberg M, Fine S (eds): Symposium on the Treatment of Diabetic Retinopathy. Washington, DC, US Department of Health, Education, and Welfare, Public Health Service No. 1890, US Government Printing Office, 1969, pp 545–53

Spalter HF: Photocoagulation of circinate maculopathy in diabetic retinopathy. Am J Ophthalmol 71:242–50, 1971

Tasman W: Retinal detachment secondary to proliferative diabetic retinopathy. Arch Ophthalmol 87:286–9, 1972

Tolentino FI, Lee PF, Schepens CL: Biomicroscopic study of vitreous cavity in diabetic retinopathy. Arch Ophthalmol 75:238–46, 1966

Retinal Vein Occlusion

Blankenship GW, Okun E: Retinal tributary vein occlusions. Arch Ophthalmol 89:363–8, 1973

Campbell CJ, Wise GN: Photocoagulation therapy of branch vein obstructions. Am J Ophthalmol 75:28–31, 1973

Chester EM: Central retinal vein occlusion. In The Ocular Fundus In Systemic Disease. Chicago, Year Book Medical Publishers, 1973, pp 116–19

Fujino T, Curtin VT, Norton EW: Experimental central retinal vein occlusion: A comparison of intraocular and extraocular occlusions. Trans Am Ophthalmol Soc 66:318–78, 1968

Gutman FA: Macular edema in branch retinal vein occlusion: Prognosis and management. Trans Am Acad Ophthalmol Otolaryngol 83:488–93, 1977

Gutman FA, Zegarra H: The natural course of temporal retinal branch vein occlusion. Trans Am Acad Ophthalmol Otolaryngol 78:178–92, 1974

Gutman FA, Zegarra H, Raver A, et al: Photocoagulation in retinal branch vein occlusion. Ann Ophthalmol 13:1359–63, 1981

Hayreh SS: Occlusion of the central retinal vessels. Br J Ophthalmol 49:626–45, 1965

Jaeger EA: Venous obstructive disease of the retina. In Duane TD (ed): Clinical Ophthalmology, vol 3. Hagerstown, MD, Harper & Row, 1978, pp 1–13

Jensen VA: Clinical studies of tributary thrombosis in the central retinal vein. Acta Ophthalmol (Suppl) 10:1–193, 1936

Kelley JS, Patz A, Schatz H: Management of retinal vein occlusion: The role of argon laser photocoagulation. Ann Ophthalmol 6:1123–34, 1974

Koyanagi Y: Die Bedeutung der Gefässkreuzung für die Entstehung der Astthrombose der retinalen Zentralvene. Klin Monatsbl Augenheilkd 81:219–31, 1928

Michels RG, Gass JDM: The natural course of retinal branch vein obstruction. Trans Am Acad Ophthalmol Otolaryngol 78:166–77, 1974

Orth DH, Patz A: Retinal branch vein occlusion. Surv Ophthalmol 22:357–76, 1978

Paton A, Rubinstein K, Smith VH: Arterial insufficiency in retinal venous occlusion. Trans Ophthalmol Soc UK 84:559–95, 1964

Rabinowicz IM, Litman S, Michaelson IC: Branch venous thrombosis: A pathological report. Trans Ophthalmol Soc UK 88:191–210, 1968

Rosen E: Fluorescein Photography of the Eye. New York, Appleton-Century-Crofts, 1969, pp 212–26

Seitz R: The Retinal Vessels: Comparative Ophthalmoscopic and Histologic Studies on Health and Diseased Eyes. St. Louis, Mosby 1964, pp 75–101

Wetzig PC: The treatment of acute branch vein occlusion by photocoagulation. Am J Ophthalmol 87:65–73, 1979

Wise GN, Dollery CT, Henkind P: Central vein occlusion. In The Retinal Circulation. New York, Harper & Row, 1971, pp 351–64

Sickle Cell Retinopathy

Edington GM, Sarkies JWR: Two cases of sickle cell anemia associated with retinal microaneurysms. Trans R Soc Trop Med Hyg 46:59–62, 1952

Goldberg MF: Natural history of untreated proliferative sickle retinopathy. Arch Ophthalmol 85:428–37, 1971

Goldberg MF: Treatment of proliferative sickle retinopathy. Trans Am Acad Ophthalmol Otolaryngol 75:532–56, 1971

Goldberg MF: Classification and pathogenesis of proliferative sickle retinopathy. Ophthalmology 71:649–65, 1971

Goldberg MF: Sickle cell retinopathy. In Duane TD (ed): Clinical Ophthalmology, vol 3. Hagerstown, MD, Harper & Row. 1976, pp 1–45

Goldberg MF: Classification and pathogenesis of proliferative sickle retinopathy. Am J Ophthalmol 71:649–65, 1971

Goldberg M, Charache S, Acacio I: Ophthalmologic manifestations of sickle cell thalassemia. Arch Intern Med 128:33–9, 1971

Goodman G, von Sallman L, Holland MG: Ocular manifestations of sickle-cell disease. Arch Ophthalmol 58:655–82, 1957

Hannon JF: Vitreous hemorrhage: Associated with sickle cell hemoglobin C disease. Am J Ophthalmol 42:707–12, 1956

Henry MD, Chapman AZ: Vitreous hemorrhage and retinopathy associated with sickle-cell disease. Am J Ophthalmol 38:204–9, 1954

Isbey EI, Tanaka KR, Clifford GO: Vitreous hemorrhage: Associated with sickle-cell trait and sickle-cell hemoglobin C disease. Am J Ophthalmol 45:870–9, 1958

Jampol LM, Goldbaum MH: Peripheral proliferative retinopathies. Surv Ophthalmol 25:1–14, 1980

Kennedy JJ, Cope CB: Intraocular lesions associated with sickle cell disease. Arch Ophthalmol 58:163–8, 1957

Lieb WA, Geeraets WJ, Guerry D III: Sickle-cell retinopathy. Acta Ophthalmol (Suppl) 58:1–45, 1959

Nagpal KC, Goldberg MF, Rabb MF: Ocular manifestations of sickle hemoglobinopathies: Surv Ophthalmol 21:391–411, 1977

Patton D: Angioid streaks and sickle cell anemia. Arch Ophthalmol 62:852–8, 1959

Romayananda N, Goldberg MF, Green WR: Histopathology of sickle cell retinopathy. Trans Am Acad Ophthalmol Otolaryngol 77:652–76, 1973

Rudd C, Evans PJ, Peeney ALP: Ocular complications in thalassemia minor. Br J Ophthalmol 37:353–8, 1953

Welch RB, Goldberg MF: Sickle-cell hemoglobin and its relation to fundus abnormality. Arch Ophthalmol 75:353–62, 1966

Retrolental Fibroplasia

Ashton N, Gardner A, Knight G: Intermittent oxygen in retrolental fibroplasia. Am J Ophthalmol 71:153–60, 1971

Ashton N, Graymore C, Pedler C: Studies on developing retinal vessels. V. Mechanism of vaso-obliteration. Br J Ophthalmol 41:449–60, 1957

Ashton N, Ward B, Serpell G: Effect of oxygen on developing retinal vessels with particular reference to the problem of retrolental fibroplasia. Br J Ophthalmol 38:397–432, 1954

Faris BM, Brockhurst RJ: Retrolental fibroplasia in the cicatricial stage. Arch Ophthalmol 82:60–5, 1969

Flynn JT, Cassady J, Essner D, et al: Fluorescein angiography in retrolental fibroplasia: Experience from 1969–1977. Ophthalmol 86: 1700–23, 1979

Friedenwald JS, Owens WC, Owens EU: Retrolental fibroplasia in premature infants. III. Pathology of the disease. Trans Am Ophthalmol Soc 49:207–34, 1951

Huggert A: Appearance of the fundus oculi in prematurely born infants treated with and without oxygen. Acta Paediatr (Uppsala) 43:327–36, 1954

King MJ: Retrolental fibroplasia: A clinical study of two hundred and thirty-eight cases. Arch Ophthalmol 43:694–711, 1950

Kingham JD: Acute retrolental fibroplasia. Arch Ophthalmol 95:39–47, 1977

Masaryk J: Fibroplasia in the vitreous. Ann Ophthalmol 4:40–6, 1972

McPherson AR, Wittner HM, Kretzer FL: Retinopathy of Prematurity: Current concepts and Controversies. Toronto, B.C. Deckner, 1986, 237 pp

Michelson PE, Patz A, Howell R: Oxygen studies in retrolental fibroplasia. Ann Ophthalmol 27:73–8, 1970

Patz A: Clinical and experimental studies on role of oxygen in retrolental fibroplasia. Trans Am Acad Ophthalmol Otolaryngol 58:45–50, 1954

Patz A: Oxygen studies in retrolental fibroplasia. IV. Clinical and experimental observations. Am J Ophthalmol 38:291–308, 1954

Patz A: Retrolental fibroplasia. Surv Ophthalmol 14:1–29, 1969

Patz A, Eastham A, Higginbotham D, Kleh T: Oxygen studies in retrolental fibroplasia: Production of microscopic changes of retrolental fibroplasia in experimental animals. Am J Ophthalmol 36:1511–22, 1953

Patz, A, Hoeck LE, De La Cruz E: Studies on effect of high oxygen administration in retrolental fibroplasia: Nursery observations. Am J Ophthalmol 35: 1248–53, 1952

Reese AB: Persistence and hyperplasia of primary vitreous: Retrolental fibroplasia –Two entities. Arch Ophthalmol 41:527–52, 1949

Reese AB, Blodi FC: Retrolental fibroplasia. Am J Ophthalmol 34:1–24, 1951

Reese AB, Payne R: Persistence and hyperplasia of the primary vitreous, tunica vasculosa lentis or retrolental fibroplasia. Trans Am Ophthalmol Soc 43:163–92, 1945

Reese AB, Stepanik J: Cicatricial stage of retrolental fibroplasia. Am J Ophthalmol 38:308–16, 1954

Tasman W: Late complications of retrolental fibroplasia. Ophthalmology 86:1724–40, 1979

Tasman W, Annesley W: Retinal detachment in the retinopathy of prematurity. Arch Ophthalmol 75:608–14, 1966

Terry TL: Extreme prematurity and fibroblastic overgrowth of persistent vascular sheath behind each crystalline lens. I. Preliminary report. Am J Ophthalmol 25:203–4, 1942

Terry TL: Fibroblastic overgrowth of persistent tunica vasculosa lentis in premature infants. II. Report of cases – Clinical aspects. Arch Ophthalmol 29:36–53, 1943

Tolentino FI, Schepens CL, Freeman HM: Vitreoretinal Disorders. Philadelphia, Saunders, 1976, pp 207–25

Zacharias L: Retrolental fibroplasia. J Pediatr 64:156–8, 1964

Inflammatory Disorders

Sarcoidosis

Chumbley LC, Kearns TP: Retinopathy of sarcoidosis. Am J Ophthalmol 73:123–31, 1972

Crick RP: Ocular sarcoidosis. Trans Ophthalmol Soc UK 75:189–206, 1955

Cross AG: Ocular sarcoidosis. Trans Ophthalmol Soc UK 75:181–7, 1955

Ferguson RH, Paris J: Sarcoidosis: Study of twenty-nine cases with a review of splenic, hepatic, mucous membrane, retinal and joint manifestations. Arch Intern Med 101:1065, 1958

Fine M, Flocks M: Bilateral acute neuroretinitis with sarcoidosis treated with cortisporin and cortisone. Arch Ophthalmol 50:358–62, 1953

Franceschetti A, Babel J: La choriorétinite en "taches de bougie" manifestation de la maladie de Besnier-Boeck. Ophthalmologica 118:701, 1949

Geeraets WJ, McNeer KW, Maxey EF, Guerry III D: Retinopathy in sarcoidosis. Acta Ophthalmol 40:492–514, 1962

Goldberg S, Newell FW: Sarcoidosis with retinal involvement. Arch Ophthalmol 32:93–6, 1944

Gould HL, Kaufman HE: Boeck's sarcoid of the ocular fundus. Am J Ophthalmol 52:633–7, 1961

Gould HL, Kaufman HE: Sarcoid of the fundus. Arch Ophthalmol 65:453–6, 1961

James DG, Anderson R, Langley DA, et al: Ocular sarcoidosis. Br J Ophthalmol 46:461–70, 1964

James DG, Neville E, Langley DA: Ocular sarcoidosis. Trans Ophthalmol Soc UK 96:133–9, 1976

Landers PN: Vitreous lesions observed in Boeck's sarcoid. Am J Ophthalmol 32:1740–1, 1949

Letocha CE, Shields JA, Goldberg RE: Retinal changes in sarcoidosis. Can J Ophthalmol 10:184–92, 1975

Levitt JM: Boeck's sarcoid with ocular localization. Arch Ophthalmol 26:358–88, 1941

MacDonald A: Boeck's sarcoid of the retina-miliary form. Trans Am Ophthalmol Soc 41:200, 1943

Maumenee AE, Zimmerman LE: Ocular aspects of sarcoidosis. Am Rev Respir Dis 84(5)Pt 2:38–44, 1961

Obenauf CD, Shaw HE, Snydor CF, Klintworth GK: Sarcoidosis and its ophthalmic manifestations. Am J Ophthalmol 86:648–55, 1978

Ohno S, Matsuda H: Association between HLA and endogenous uveitis. In Acta: Henkind P (ed): 24th International Congress of Ophthalmology. Philadelphia, Lippincott, 1982, pp 558–60

Harada's Syndrome
(Vogt-Koyanagi-Harada's Syndrome)

Harada Y: (A clinical study of nonsupportive choroiditis (acute diffuse choroiditis). Nippon Ganka Gakkai Zasshi (Acta Soc Ophthalmol Jpn) 30:356–78, 1926

Koyanagi Y: Dysakosis, Alopecia und Poliosisbei Schwerer Uveitis nicht traumatischen Ursprungs. Klin Monatsbl Augenheilkd 82:194–211, 1929

Ohno S, Char DH, Kimura SJ, O'Connor GR: Vogt-Koyanagi-Harada syndrome. Am J Ophthalmol 83: 735–40, 1977

Pattison EM: Uveomeningoencephalitic syndrome (Vogt-Koyanagi-Harada). Arch Neurol 12:197–205, 1965

Perry HD, Font RL: Clinical and histopathologic observations in severe Vogt-Koyanagi-Harada syndrome. Am J Ophthalmol 83:242–54, 1977

Rogell G: Infections and inflammatory diseases. In Duane TD(ed): Clinical Ophthalmology, vol 3. Philadelphia, Harper & Row, 1981, pp 1–24

Shimizu K: Harada's, Behcet's, Vogt-Koyanagi syndromes: Are they clinical entities? Trans Am Acad Ophthalmol Otolaryngol 77:281–90, 1973

Suguira S: Vogt-Koyanagi-Harada disease. Jpn J Ophthalmol 22:9–35, 1978

Synder DA, Tessler HH: Vogt-Koyanagi-Harada syndrome. Am J Ophthalmol 90:69–75, 1980

Yoshioka H: Fluorescence fundus angiographic findings in early stages of Harada's syndrome. Acta Soc Ophthalmol Jpn 72:2298–306, 1968

Pars Planitis (Peripheral Uveitis)

Aaberg TM, Cesarz TJ, Flinkinger RR: Treatment of peripheral uveoretinitis by cryotherapy. Am J Ophthalmol 73:685–8, 1973

Brockhurst RJ, Schepens CL, Okamura ID: Uveitis I. Gonioscopy. Am J Ophthalmol 42: 545–54, 1956

Brockhurst RJ, Schepens CL, Okamura ID: Uveitis II. Peripheral uveitis: Clinical description, complications and differential diagnosis. Am J Ophthalmol 49:1257–66, 1960

Brockhurst RJ, Schepens CL, Okamura ID: Uveitis III. Peripheral uveitis: Pathogenesis, etiology and treatment. Am J Ophthalmol 51:19–26, 1961

Brockhurst RJ, Schepens CL: Uveitis IV: Peripheral uveitis: The complication of retinal detachment. Arch Ophthalmol 80:747–53, 1968

Pruett RC, Brockhurst RJ, Letts N: Fluorescein angiography of peripheral uveitis. Am J Ophthalmol 77:448–53, 1974

Schepens CL: Examination of the ora serrata region: Its clinical significance. In: Acta: 16th Concilium Ophthalmologicum, Britannia, 1950. London, British Medical Association, 1951, vol 2, pp 1384–93

Schepens, CL: L'inflammation de la région de l' "ora serrata" et ses séquelles. Bull Mem Soc Fr Ophtalmol 63:113–25, 1950

Schepens CL: Retinal Detachment and Allied Diseases, vol 2. Philadelphia, Saunders, 1983, pp 672–82

Smith RE, Godfrey SA, Kimura SJ: Chronic cyclitis I. Course and visual prognosis. Trans Am Acad Ophthalmol Otolaryngol 77:760–8, 1973

Smith RE, Godfrey SA, Kimura SJ: Complications of chronic cyclitis. Am J Ophthalmol 82:277–82, 1976

Choroidal Detachments

Bietti GB: Hemorrhagic choroidal detachments. In McPherson A (ed): New and Controversial Aspects of Retinal Detachment. New York, Harper & Row, 1968, pp 471–2

Brav SS: Serous choroidal detachment. Surv Ophthalmol 6:395–415, 1961

Chignell AH: Choroidal detachment following retinal detachment surgery without drainage of subretinal fluid. Am J Ophthalmol 73:860–2, 1972

Gottlieb F: Combined choroidal and retinal detachment. Arch Ophthalmol 88:481–6, 1972

Hawkins WR, Schepens CL: Choroidal detachment and retinal surgery: A clinical and experimental study. Am J Ophthalmol 62:812–19, 1966

Schepens CL: Importance of choroidal detachment in fundus diagnosis. Am J Ophthalmol 51:333–4, 1961

Schepens CL: Retinal Detachment and Allied Diseases, vol 2. Philadelphia, Saunders, 1983, 1003–11

Seelenfreund MH, Kraushar MF, Schepens CL, et al: Choroidal detachment associated with primary retinal detachment. Arch Ophthalmol 91:254–8, 1974

Tolentino FI, Brockhurst RJ: Unilateral scleral icterus due to choroidal hemorrhage. Arch Ophthalmol 70:358–60, 1963

Choroidal Effusion Syndrome

Brockhurst RJ: Nanophthalmos with uveal effusion: A new clinical entity. Trans Am Ophthalmol Soc 72:371–403, 1974

Fogle JA, Green WR: Ciliochoroidal effusion. In Duane TD (ed): Clinical Ophthalmology, vol 4. Philadelphia, Harper & Row, 1981, pp 1–32

McDonald PR, de la Paz Jr V, Sarin LK: Nonrhegmatogenous retinal separation associated with choroidal detachment. Trans Am Ophthalmol Soc 62:226–47, 1964

Schepens CL: Retinal Detachment and Allied Diseases, vol 2. Philadelphia, Saunders, 1983, pp 731–7

Schepens CL, Brockhurst RJ: Uveal effusion. I. Clinical picture. Arch Ophthalmol 70:189–201, 1963

Pigmentary Tumors of the Peripheral Retina

Choroidal Nevi

Ganley LP, Comstock GW: Benign nevi and malignant melanomas of the choroid. Am J Ophthalmol 76:19–25, 1973

Gass JDM: Problems in the differential diagnosis of choroidal nevi and malignant melanomas. The 33rd Edward Jackson Memorial Lecture. Am J Ophthalmol 83:299–323, 1977

Naumann G, Hellner KM, Naumann LR: Pigmented nevi of the choroid. Clinical study of the secondary changes in the overlying tissues. Trans Am Acad Ophthalmol Otolaryngol 75:110–23, 1971

Pro M, Shields JA, Tomer TL: Serous detachment of the forea associated with presumed choroidal nevi. Arch Ophthalmol 96:1374–7, 1978

Shields JA: Tumors of the uveal tract. In

Duane TD (ed): Clinical Ophthalmology, vol 4. Philadelphia, Harper & Row, 1981, pp 1–13

Shields JA, Rodrigues MM, Sarin LK, et al: Lipofuscin pigment over benign and malignant choroidal tumors. Trans Am Acad Ophthalmol Otolaryngol 81:871–81, 1976

Tamler E: A clinical study of choroidal nevi. A follow-up report. Arch Ophthalmol 84:29–32, 1970

Tamler E, Maumanee AE: A clinical study of choroidal nevi. Arch Ophthalmol 62:196–202, 1959

Waltman DD, Gitter KA, Yannuzzi L, et al: Choroidal neovascularization associated with choroidal nevi. Am J Ophthalmol 85:704–10, 1978

Congenital Hypertrophy of the Retinal Pigment Epithelium (CHRPE)

Boldrey EE, Schwartz A: Enlargement of congenital hypertrophy of the pigment epithelium. Am J Ophthalmol 94:64–6, 1982

Buettner H: Congenital hypertrophy of the retinal pigment epithelium. Am J Ophthalmol 79:177–90, 1975

Cleary PE, Gregor Z, Bird AC: Retinal vascular changes in congenital hypertrophy of the retinal pigment epithelium. Br J Ophthalmol 60:499–503, 1976

Kurz GH, Zimmerman LE: Vagaries of the retinal pigment epithelium. Int Ophthalmol Clin 2:441–64, 1962

Norris JL, Cleasby GW: An unusual case of congenital hypertrophy of the retinal pigment epithelium. Arch Ophthalmol 94:1910–11, 1976

Purcell JJ, Shields JA: Hypertrophy with hyperpigmentation of the retinal pigment epithelium. Arch Ophthalmol 93:1122–6, 1975

Reese AB, Jones IS: Benign melanomas of the retinal pigment epithelium. Am J Ophthalmol 42:207–12, 1956

Congenital Grouped Pigmentation (Bear Tracks)

Forsius H, Eriksson A, Nuutlia A, et al: A genetic study of three rare retinal disorders: Dystrophia retinal dysacusis syndrome, X-chromosomal retinoschisis and grouped pigments of the retina. Birth Defects 7:83–98, 1971

Hoeg H: Die gruppierte Pigmentation des Augengrundes. Klin Monatsbl Augenheilkd 49:49–77, 1911

Legrand MJ, Hervouet F, Baron A, et al:

Pigmentation groupée de la rétine. Bull Soc Ophthalmol Fr 64:313–15, 1964

Mauthner L: Lehrbuch der Ophthalmoskopie. Wien, Ed. Fendler, 1868, p 338

Shields JA, Tso MO: Congenital grouped pigmentation of the retina. Arch Ophthalmol 93:1153–5, 1975

Stephenson S: A peculiar form of retinal pigmentation. Trans Ophthalmol Soc UK 11:77, 1891

Waardenberg PJ, Franceschetti A, Klein D: Genetics of and Ophthalmology, vol I. Springfield, IL, Charles C Thomas, 1961, p 548

Metastatic Tumors to the Choroid

Albert DM, Rubenstein RA, Scheie HG: Tumor metastasis to the eye. Part I. Incidence in two-hundred and thirteen adult patients with generalized malignancy. Am J Ophthalmol 63:723–6, 1967

Bloch RS, Gartner S: The incidence of ocular metastatic carcinoma. Arch Ophthalmol 85:673–5, 1971

Davis DL, Robertson DM: Fluorescein angiography of metastatic choroidal tumors. Arch Ophthalmol 89:97–9, 1973

Ferry AP: Lesions mistaken for malignant melanoma of the posterior uvea. Arch Ophthalmol 72:463–9, 1964

Ferry AP: The biological behavior and pathological features of carcinoma metastatic to the eye and orbit. Trans Am Ophthalmol Soc 71:373–425, 1973

Ferry AP, Font RL: Carcinoma metastatic to the eye and orbit. A clinicopathologic study of two-hundred and twenty-seven cases. Arch Ophthalmol 92:276–86, 1974

Fishman M, Tomaszewski M, Kuwabara T: Malignant melanoma of the skin metastatic to the eye. Arch Ophthalmol 9:1309–11, 1976

Gass JDM: Differential Diagnosis of Intraocular Tumors. A Stereoscopic Presentation. St. Louis, Mosby, 1974, pp 140–158

Gitter K, Meyer D, Sarin L, et al: Fluorescein angiography of metastatic choroid tumors. Arch Ophthalmol 89:97–9, 1973

Godtfredsen E: On the frequency of secondary carcinomas in the choroid. Acta Ophthalmol 22:304, 1944

Greear JN: Metastatic carcinoma of the eye. Am J Ophthalmol 33:1015–25, 1950

Greer C: Choroidal carcinoma metastatic from the male breast. Br J Ophthalmol 38:312–15, 1954

Jaeger EA, Frayer WC, Southard ME, et al: Effect of radiation therapy on metastatic choroidal tumors. Trans Am Acad Ophthalmol Otolaryngol 75:94–101, 1971

Reese AB: Tumors of the Eye, 3rd ed. Hagerstown, MD, Harper & Row, 1976, pp 424–31

Shields J: Metastatic tumors to and from the eye. In Croll M, Brady L, Wallner R (eds): Nuclear Ophthalmology. New York, Wiley, 1976, pp 151–60

Usher C: Cases of metastatic carcinoma of the choroid and iris. Br J Ophthalmol 7:10, 1923

Choroidal Melanomas

Callender GR: Malignant melanotic tumors of the eye, a study of histologic types in one hundred and eleven cases. Trans Am Acad Ophthalmol Otolaryngol 36:131, 1931

Callender GR, Wilder HC, Ash JE: Five hundred malignant melanomas of the choroid and ciliary body followed five years or longer. Am J Ophthalmol 25:962–7, 1942

Coleman DJ: Reliability of ocular trauma diagnosis with ultrasound. Trans Am Acad Ophthalmol Otolaryngol 77:677–86, 1973

Davidorf H, Lang JR: The natural history of malignant melanoma of the choroid: Small vs. large tumors. Trans Am Acad Ophthalmol Otolaryngol 79:310–20, 1975

Ferry AP: Lesions mistaken for malignant melanomas of the posterior uvea: A clinicopathologic analysis of one hundred cases with ophthalmoscopically visible lesions. Arch Ophthalmol 72: 463–9, 1964

Font RL, Zimmerman LE, Armaly MF: The nature of the orange pigment over a choroidal melanoma: Histochemical and electron microscopic observations. Arch Ophthalmol 91:359–62, 1974

Gass JDM: Hemorrhage into the vitreous, a presenting manifestation of malignant melanoma of the choroid. Arch Ophthalmol 69:778–9, 1963

Gass JDM: Problems in the differential diagnosis of choroidal nevi and malignant melanomas. The 33rd Jackson Memorial Lecture. Am J Ophthalmol 83:299–323, 1977

Hedges TR, Leopold IH: Parallel retinal folds. Their significance in orbital space taking lesions. Arch Ophthalmol 62:353–5, 1959

Jacobiec FA: Ocular and Adnexal Tumors. Birmingham, AL, Aesculapius, 1978

McLean IW, Foster WD, Zimmerman LE: Prognostic factors in small malignant melanomas of choroid and ciliary body. Arch Ophthalmol 95:48–58, 1977

Newell FW: Choroidal folds. Am J Ophthalmol 75:930–42, 1973

Reese AB: Tumors of the Eye, 3rd ed. Hagerstown, MD, Harper & Row, 1976, pp 193–223

Shields JA: Current approaches to the diagnosis and management of choroidal melanomas. Surv Ophthalmol 21:443–63, 1977

Shields JA, Hagler WS, Federman JL, et al: The significance of the 32-P uptake test in the diagnosis of posterior uveal melanoma. Trans Am Acad Ophthalmol Otolaryngol 79:297–306, 1975

Shields JA, McDonald PR: Improvements in the diagnosis of posterior uveal melanomas. Arch Ophthalmol 91:259–64, 1974

Shields JA, Rodrigues MM, Sarin LK, et al: Lipofuscin pigment over benign and malignant choroidal tumors. Trans Am Acad Ophthalmol Otolaryngol 81:871–81, 1976

Shields JA, Zimmerman LE: Lesions simulating malignant melanoma of the posterior uvea. Arch Ophthalmol 89:466–71, 1973

Zimmerman LE: Problems in the diagnosis of malignant melanomas of the choroid and ciliary body. Am J Ophthalmol 75:917–29, 1970

Zimmerman LE, McLean IW: Changing concepts in the prognosis and management of small malignant melanomas of the choroid. In Peyman CA, Apple DS, Sanders DR (eds): Intraocular Tumors. New York, Appleton-Century-Crofts, 1977, pp 63–74

Retinitis Pigmentosa

Berson FL, Gouras P, Gunkel RD: Rod responses in retinitis pigmentosa dominantly inherited. Arch Ophthalmol 80:58–67, 1968

Berson FL: Light deprivation for early retinitis pigmentosa. Arch Ophthalmol 85:521–9, 1971

Bloome MA, Garcia CA: Rod and cone dystrophies. In Bloome MA, Garcia CA: Manual of Retinal and Choroidal Dystrophies. New York, Appleton-Century-Crofts, 1982, Chapter 5. pp 39–58

Bonavolontar A: La biomicroscopia del vitreo nella retinite pigmentosa. Ann Ottal 77:15–20, 1951

Carr RF: Primary retinal degenerations. In Duane TD (ed): Clinical Ophthalmology, vol 3. New York, Harper & Row, 1981, pp 1–19

Deutman AF: Rod-cone dystrophy: Primary, hereditary, pigmentary retinopathy, retinitis pigmentosa. In Archer DB (ed): Krill's Hereditary Retinal and Choroidal Diseases, vol 2: Clinical Characteristics. Hagerstown, MD, Harper & Row, 1977, pp 429–536

Dewar AJ, Reading HW: The biochemical aspects of retinitis pigmentosa. Int J Biochem 6:615–41, 1975

Donders FC: Beiträge zur pathologischen Anatomie des Auges; 2) Pigmentbildung in der Netzhaut. Graefes Arch Ophthalmol 3:139–50, 1857

Francois J: Heredity in Ophthalmology. St. Louis, Mosby, 1961, pp 441–86

Green WR: Retina. In Spencer WH: Ophthalmic Pathology: An Atlas and Textbook, vol. 2, 3rd ed. Philadelphia, Saunders, 1985, pp 1210–21

Liebreich R: Abkunft aus Ehen unter Blutsverwandten als Grund von Retinitis pigmentosa. Dtsch Klin 13:53–5, 1861

Lucas DR: Retinitis pigmentosa. Br J Ophthalmol 40:14–23, 1956

Merin S, Auerbach A: Retinitis pigmentosa. Surv Ophthalmol 20:303–46, 1976

Nishida S, Mizuno K: Electron microscopy of the pigmentary degeneration of the human retina. Acta Soc Ophthalmol Jpn 75:1779–89, 1971

Pillat A: Hintere Glaskörperabhebung bei Retinitis Pigmentosa. Z Augenheilkd. 61:140, 1927

Pruett RC: Retinitis pigmentosa: A biomicroscopical study of irrteous abnormalities. Arch Ophthalmol 93:603–08, 1975

Reiger H: Über die Bedeutung der Aderhautveränderungen für die Entstehung der Glaskörperabhebung. Arch Ophthalmol 136:119–65, 1936

Szamier RB, Berson DL: Retinal ultrastructure in advanced retinitis pigmentosa. Invest Ophthalmol 16:947–62, 1977

Van Trigt AC: De cogspiegel. Thesis. Utrecht, Ned. Lancot (3d ser.) 2:492, 1853

Von Graefe A: Über die Untersuchung des Gesichtsfeldes bei Amblyopischen Affektionen. Graefes Arch Ophthalmol 2:263–4, 282–4, 1856

Developmental Disorders

Colobomas of Retina and Choroid

Coats G: The pathology of coloboma at the nerve entrance. London Ophthalmol Hosp Rep 17:178, 1908

Francois J: Colobomatous malformations of the ocular globe. Int Ophthalmol Clin 8:797–816, 1968

Freeman HM: Congenital retinal diseases. In Tasman WS (ed): Retinal diseases in children. New York, Harper & Row, 1971, pp 4–5

Hird B: An exhaustive treatise on the various colobomas. Ophthalmol Rev 31:162, 1912

Hovland KR, Schepens CL, Freeman HM: Developmental giant retinal tears associated with lens coloboma. Arch Ophthalmol 80:325–31, 1968

Jesberg DO, Schepens CL: Retinal detachment associated with coloboma of the choroid. Arch Ophthalmol 65:163–73, 1961

Pagon RA: Ocular coloboma. Surv Ophthalmol 25:223–6, 1981

Long-Standing Retinal Detachments

Intraocular Fibrosis

Chignell AH: Retinal Detachment Surgery. Berlin, Springer-Verlag, 1980, pp 36–7

Cibis P: Vitreoretinal Pathology and Surgery in Retinal Detachment. St. Louis, Mosby, 1965, pp 77–9

Clarkson JG, Green WR, Massof D: A histopathologic review of 168 cases of preretinal membrane. Am J Ophthalmol 84:1–24, 1977

Constable IF, Oguri M, Chesney CM, et al: Platelet-induced vitreous membrane formation. Invest Ophthalmol 12:680–5, 1973

Constable IJ, Swann DS: Biological vitreous substitutes. Inflammatory response in normal and altered animal eyes. Arch Ophthalmol 88:544–8, 1972

Constable IJ, Tolentino FI, Donovan RH, Schepens CL: Clinico-pathologic correlation of vitreous membranes. In Pruett RC, Regan CDJ (eds): Retina Congress. New York, Appleton-Century-Crofts, 1974, pp 245–57

Foos RY: Anatomic and pathologic aspects of the vitreous body. Trans Am Acad Ophthalmol Otolaryngol 77:171–83, 1973

Gloor BP: Cellular proliferation on the vit-

reous surface after photocoagulation. Graefes Arch Klin Exp Ophthalmol 178:99–113, 1969

Hogan MJ, Zimmerman LE: Ophthalmic Pathology. Philadelphia, Saunders, 1962, pp 549–68

Jalk AE, Marcos PA, Schepens CL, Azzolini C, Duncan JE, Trempe CL: Surgical treatments of proliferative vitreoretinopathy. Arch Ophthalmol 102:1135–39, 1984

Lam KW, Ashrafzadeh T, Lee CB: Vitreous membranes. Induction in rabbits by intravitreous leukocyte injections. Arch Ophthalmol 88:655–8, 1972

Laqua H, Machemer R: Glial cell proliferation in retinal detachment (massive periretinal proliferation). Am J Ophthalmol 80:602–18, 1975

Laqua H, Machemer R: Clinico-pathological correlation in massive periretinal proliferation. Am J Ophthalmol 80:913–29, 1975

Leber T: Die Krankheiten der Netzhaut. In Graefe A von, Saemisch ET (eds): Handbuch der Augenheilkunde, vol 3 (2). Leipzig, Englemann, 1915, pp 1501–03

Machemer R: Experimental retinal detachment in the owl monkey. 2. Histology of the retina and pigment epithelium. Am J Ophthalmol 66:396–410, 1968

Machemer R: Pathogenesis and classification of massive periretinal proliferation. Br J Ophthalmol 62:737–47, 1978

Machemer R, Laqua H: Pigment epithelium proliferation in retinal detachment. (Massive periretinal proliferation). Am J Ophthalmol 80:1–23, 1975

Machemer R, Van Horn D, Aaberg TM: Pigment epithelial proliferation in human retinal detachment with massive periretinal proliferation. Am J Ophthalmol 85:181–91, 1978

Magusar MA, Lam KW, Tolentino FL, Liu HS: Lymphocyte-induced vitreous membranes: A comparative study with leukocyte and platelet-induced vitreous membranes. Invest Ophthalmol 14:240–3, 1975

Mandelcorn MS, Machemer R, Fineberg E, Hersch SB: Proliferation and metaplasia of intravitreal retinal pigment epithelium cell autotransplants. Am J Ophthalmol 80:227–37, 1975

Mueller-Jensen K, Machemer R, Azarnia R: Autotransplantation of retinal pigment epithelium in intravitreal diffusion chambers. Am J Ophthalmol 80:530–7, 1975

Parsons JH: The Pathology of the Eye.

Histology. London, Hodder and Stroughton, 1905, pp 542–600

Regnault FR: Vitreous hemorrhage: An experimental study. I. A macroscopic and isotopic study of the evolution of whole blood and hemoglobin. Arch Ophthalmol 83:458–65, 1970

Regnault FR: Vitreous hemorrhage. II. Hemoglobin degradation. Arch Ophthalmol 83:466–9, 1970

Regnault FR: Vitreous hemorrhage. III. Experimental degeneration of the rabbit retina induced by hemoglobin injection into the vitreous. Arch Ophthalmol 83:470–3, 1970

The Retina Society Terminology Committee: The classification of retinal detachment with proliferative vitreoretinopathy. Ophthalmology 90:121–25, 1983

Roth AM, Foos RY: Surface structure of the optic nerve head. I. Epipapillary membranes. Am J Ophthalmol 74:977–85, 1972

Schepens CL: Retinal Detachment and Allied Diseases, vol 2. Philadelphia, Saunders, 1983, pp 177–213.

Smith T: Pathologic findings after retina surgery. In Schepens CL (ed): Importance of the Vitreous Body in Retina Surgery with Special Emphasis on Reoperations. St. Louis, Mosby, 1960, pp 61–93

Teng CC: Discussion of Smith TR: Pathologic findings after retinal surgery. In Schepens CL (ed): Importance of the Vitreous Body in Retina Surgery with Special Emphasis on Reoperations. St. Louis, Mosby, 1960, pp 76–91

Tolentino FI, Schepens CL, Freeman HM: Vitreoretinal Disorders. Diagnosis and Management. Philadelphia, Saunders, 1976, pp 471–89

Van Horn DL, Aaberg TM, Machemer R, Fenzl R: Glial cell proliferation in human retinal detachment with massive periretinal proliferation. Am J Ophthalmol 84:383–93, 1977

Yanoff M, Fine BS: Ocular Pathology. Hagerstown, MD, Harper & Row, 1975, pp 455–562

Zinn K, Constable I, Schepens CL: The fine structure of human vitreous membranes. In Freeman HM, Hirose T, Schepens CL (eds): Vitreous Surgery and Advances in Fundus Diagnosis Treatment. New York, Appleton-Century-Crofts, 1977, pp 34–49

Demarcation Lines

Benson WE, Nantawan P, Morse PH: Characteristics and prognosis of retinal detachments with demarcation lines. Am J Ophthalmol 84:641–4, 1977

Hogan M, Zimmerman LE: Ophthalmic Pathology. Philadelphia, Saunders, 1962, pp 549–68

Schepens CL: Diagnostic and prognostic factors as found in preoperative examination. (Symposium: Retinal Detachment). Trans Am Acad Ophthalmol Otolaryngol 56:398–418, 1952

Retinal Cysts

Chignell AH: Retinal Detachment Surgery. Berlin, Springer-Verlag, 1980, pp 36–7

Hagler WS, North AW: Intraretinal macrocysts and retinal detachment. Trans Am Acad Ophthalmol Otolaryngol 71:442–54, 1967

Ruiz RS: Hemorrhagic macrocyst of the retina. Arch Ophthalmol 83:588–90, 1970

Schepens CL: Retinal Detachment and Allied Diseases, vol 1. Philadelphia, Saunders, 1983, pp 214–32

Schepens CL, Tolentino F, McMeel JW: Diagnostic and prognostic factors as found in preoperative examination. In Pischel D (ed): Retinal Detachment, 2nd ed. Rochester, MN, American Academy of Ophthalmology and Otolaryngology, 1965, pp 51–85

Shrinkage of Retinal Tear Flaps and Opercula

Byer NE: The Peripheral Retina in Profile. A Stereoscopic Atlas. Torrance, CA, Criterion Press, 1982, 159 pp

Rutnin U, Schepens CL: Fundus appearance in normal eyes. IV. Retinal breaks and other findings. Am J Ophthalmol 64:1063–78, 1967

Spencer LM, Straatsma BR, Foos RY: Tractional degenerations of the peripheral retina. In New Orleans Academy of Ophthalmology: Symposium of the Retina and Retinal Surgery. St. Louis, Mosby, 1969, pp 103–27

Index

Page numbers in italics refer to figure plates.